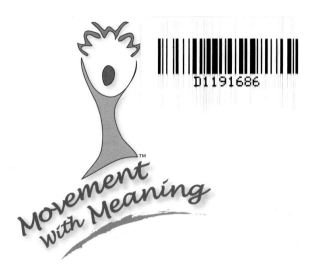

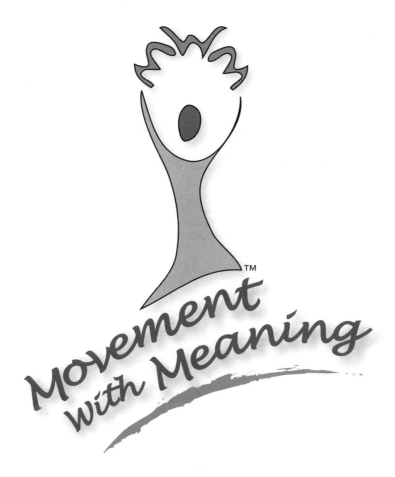

TM

A Multisensory Program
for Individuals with
Early-Stage Alzheimer's Disease

by

Barbara Larsen, M.A. Ed.

edited by

L.G. Mansfield

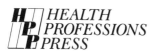

HEALTH
PROFESSIONS
PRESS

Baltimore • London • Sydney

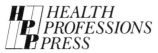

HEALTH PROFESSIONS PRESS

Health Professions Press, Inc.
Post Office Box 10624
Baltimore, Maryland 21285-0624

www.healthpropress.com

Typeset by International Graphic Services of New Jersey, Inc., Newtown, Pennsylvania.
Manufactured in the United States of America by
Versa Press, Inc., East Peoria, Illinois.

Note to readers: All exercise involves some risk. Before beginning any new physical activity, older people should consult their physicians. This book is sold without warranties of any kind, expressed or implied, and the publisher and authors disclaim any liability, loss, or damage caused by the contents of this book.

Photographs by Gail Lipson and used by permission of the photographer and featured participants.

Movement with Meaning™ and its logo are trademarks owned by Barbara Larsen.
Logo design by Patricia Montijo.

Library of Congress Cataloging-in-Publication Data

Larsen, Barbara.
   Movement with meaning : a multisensory program for individuals with early-stage Alzheimer's disease / by Barbara Larsen ; edited by L.G. Mansfield.
      p.   cm.
   Includes bibliographical references.
   ISBN-13: 978-1-932529-14-2 (pbk.)
   ISBN-10: 1-932529-14-4 (pbk.)
   1. Alzheimer's disease—Patients—Rehabilitation—Popular works.
   2. Alzheimer's disease—Patients—Recreation—Popular works.   I. Title.
   RC523.L37 2006
   616.8'31062—dc22   2005033186

British Library Cataloguing in Publication data are available from the British Library.

For the women who raised me:

Eugenia

Angelina

Flora

Ever present, everywhere, at all times

Contents

About the Author

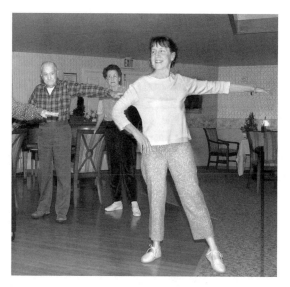

Barbara Larsen, M.A. Ed., has been working in the field of dementia care since 1985. Movement with Meaning™ is the culmination of her practical, hands-on approach to providing a multisensory program for people who have early-stage Alzheimer's disease.

Over the past 2 decades, Barbara's extensive experience has encompassed working with individuals with dementia, family caregivers, and health care professionals in a variety of settings. As an educator, director, and consultant she has brought her expertise to adult day care facilities, hospitals, residential care facilities, county and state agencies, research universities, community organizations, hospice programs, and the private sector. She has written numerous articles and presented Movement with Meaning at the annual conferences of organizations such as the Greater Sacramento Area Chapter of the Alzheimer's Association and the American Society on Aging. Since 1988, Barbara has been an education and family consultant for Del Oro Caregiver Resource Center (Carmichael, California), a statewide nonprofit organization serving the needs of family caregivers.

Preface
Beatrice's Story

"We want people to feel with us more than to act for us."
—George Eliot

In the late 1980s the senior center of our local rural community in northern California received grant funding for an adult social day care program. In my early 40s, I had changed my career as a special education teacher to a communication and language specialist in the field of dementia care, and now I was program director of the center. I was excited about my new position, especially because it gave me an opportunity to work in an environment that allowed me to apply, in a broader arena, the multisensory techniques I had developed.

One of my first encounters was with Beatrice. Beatrice had gotten lost a few times while walking to her local grocery store, and concerned neighbors alerted her daughter. When she began showing more signs of early-stage Alzheimer's disease, her daughter invited Beatrice to live with her in a small community in the Sierra foothills. After the move, the daughter noticed that Beatrice was becoming more withdrawn, unlike the lively extrovert she had always been. She also was having difficulty managing her finances; for example, she would forget to pay her telephone bill or she would put two checks in a billing envelope. These behaviors were unlike Beatrice, who had been an organized, methodical person.

After a telephone interview with Beatrice's daughter, I made an appointment for the two women to visit the day care center. On the day of the appointment, I was talking with a volunteer when the front door flew open with the force of a whirlwind and Beatrice swept into the activity room. Her eyes were clear and alert as she scanned her surroundings. Then, as though sparks ignited from her combustible imagination, Beatrice started to sing "Santa Lucia"—with great enthusiasm! The roomful of people stopped what they were doing and watched her with fascination. Beatrice had arrived!

I walked toward her with my hand extended in welcome. With a big crescent moon grin she grabbed it, pulled me closer to her, and patted my back. Although Beatrice's grip was hard, her fingers were long and fine. Her face was smooth, with a luster that gave her an air of nobility. Her enthusiasm was contagious, and we all laughed out loud together.

I invited Beatrice's daughter to tour the day care facility with our activities director while Beatrice and I went to another room. I was curious to see whether she had the ability to contain her gregarious energy. Would she be able to settle down enough to enjoy the center?

Beatrice and I sat next to each other at a long metal table. I began to massage her back gently while she hummed an unrecognizable tune. I focused my breathing in rhythm with her inhalation and exhalation. Slowly she turned her head and made eye contact with me. She was calm and relaxed. I took out a sheet of butcher paper and placed it on the table. With a large felt pen I wrote 11 letters randomly from the alphabet and Beatrice identified 7 of them correctly. I asked her if she would like to come to the day care center. She nodded and said, "Yes, sweetie."

Beatrice liked being with the other participants. During the morning session, participants were divided into small groups to focus on addressing individual interests and functional levels. Beatrice was in the music therapy circle. She remembered songs from her childhood and early adult years, and she always sang with uninhibited gusto and purpose.

In the afternoons we were fortunate to enjoy the bountiful talents of members of our community who volunteered their time with music, poetry, pet therapy, and art appreciation. On one such afternoon the activity was to create a collage of favorite plants and flowers. While the participants were engaged in the activity, Beatrice flipped through a *Better Homes and Gardens* magazine at a rapid pace, seemingly not interested in the project.

Suddenly she stopped. After studying a page for a couple of minutes, she waved me over. The photograph she pointed to showed a nontraditional landscape garden with a variety of plants and flowers growing close together and a small path leading to a white wooden gate. The words written on the top of the page read "Carefully Choreographed Chaos." Beatrice read the words out loud. I bent over her and asked, "Is this what it feels like to have Alzheimer's?" As Beatrice leaned back in her chair, she let out a "yeah" and gave me a light swat on my behind with the flat of her hand.

I tore the page from the magazine and pinned it on our bulletin board, thinking to myself, "Someday this will be a chapter in a book."

Acknowledgments

All along the way, from the inception of Movement with Meaning™ until the present time, I have been supported and encouraged by some wonderful and extraordinary people.

In bringing the multisensory aspects of the program together, Katie Carter, yoga instructor and sister pilgrim, assisted me with a variety of ideas for the chair and standing poses. *Namaste!*

The first Movement with Meaning class was held at the Lutz Adult Day Health Care Center. I am indebted to Liz Mantel, executive director, and Francine Novak, both of whom were very supportive and generous in providing a calm, nurturing environment.

As the program evolved, my colleagues and dear friends Janet Claypoole, executive director, and Michelle Nevins, education coordinator, both of Del Oro Caregiver Resource Center, demonstrated their faith in the program and in me by letting it come to fruition, organically and in its own time. They have endorsed and promoted Movement with Meaning by sponsoring workshops and seminars, including the workshop sponsored for the annual conference of the Greater Sacramento Area Chapter of the Alzheimer's Association in 2001 and the American Society on Aging's annual conference in 2002. I wrap my invisible arms around them.

I am eternally grateful to my friend, literary mentor, and editor L.G. (Elle) Mansfield for her immeasurable patience and kindness in providing a framework from which I could develop Movement with Meaning from an in-service model to a completed manuscript. Elle was akin to a midwife providing careful attention to detail while holding me in unwavering support, bringing this book to birth. She is a true kindred spirit. *Con tanto amore!*

To Joanna Robinson I give a loving, heartfelt thank-you for her expertise in the final editing of the book proposal and the completed manuscript. Joanna brings much joy and grace to my life. I am very appreciative of the time Vicki L. Schmall, gerontology and training specialist, spent reading the manuscript and offering helpful comments and suggestions. And I owe a special debt to Renee Chevraux, whose idea for and compilation of a qualitative study of memory-impaired residents at Highgate Senior Living in a month-long Movement with Meaning class proved invaluable. Renee's dedication and compassion in the field of Alzheimer's care is awe inspiring.

Lynn Jefferson, Anne Menzies, Darylann Ogden, and the staff of Highgate Senior Living embraced me, as well as Movement with Meaning, with their continued support not only of the qualitative study and photography sessions with the residents but also of an ongoing class that continues to this day. Through them I have experienced the warmth of friendship and the gift of community.

For assisting me in finding research citations for Movement with Meaning, I am very grateful to the four reference librarians in my community: Martha Kinne, Tonya Kraft, Katrin Olafsson, and Mary Ann Trygg. I appreciated their welcoming smiles and caring attention each time I asked for yet another reference in support of my work.

To Alison Pomatto, I give a special thank-you. Her knowledge of publishing houses guided me in acquiring permission for the various quotations, poems, and songs throughout the book.

Gail Lipson, photographer extraordinaire, embraced and embodied the text of Movement with Meaning. Gail's meaningful and careful consideration for each participant is made evident by the richness in every photograph. The essence of Movement with Meaning is grounded in the photographs. I thank my lucky stars for our friendship.

Patricia Montijo, artist and teacher, designed the logo for Movement with Meaning. Her design encapsulated its breadth and spectrum in a symbol that unifies the program with an essential and unique identity. *Te amo, mi amiga!*

While this book is a creation of my many years of experience in working with individuals with early-stage Alzheimer's disease, I would like to give a warm thank-you to Mary Magnus, Amy Kopperude, Trish Byrnes, and Erin Geoghegan for working with me in mutual harmony and respect during the sometimes challenging demands of publication.

To my daughter Claire, for her generous and unflagging support, I am especially grateful. She stood by and cheered me on at every new development of Movement with Meaning. Claire's presence in my life reaffirms how truly blessed I am.

To my husband Bill I am very grateful for his ever-constant love and loyalty. His insightful and intuitive nature gave me room to explore, formulate, and weave together the medley of multisensory activities that evolved into Movement with Meaning. I am indeed fortunate to have him for my spiritual partner.

At the heart of Movement with Meaning are the participants. They sustained me through their courage and their willingness to allow me to witness their journey with Alzheimer's disease. Their trusting, adventuresome, and humorous spirit continues to enrich each and every class. I thank these dear friends from the bottom of my heart!

Introduction
New Horizons
in Alzheimer's Care

We are on the brink of a new horizon in Alzheimer's care. As research propels us forward, we are uncovering facts about the disease that will forever alter the treatment process.

Nearly three quarters of a century have transpired between the discovery of the disease by Dr. Alois Alzheimer in 1906 and the early 1980s, when we achieved our first understanding of the tangles and plaques in the brains of people experiencing Alzheimer's disease. Before 1980, pathologists and geneticists examining such brains during an autopsy would see wads of sticky debris and neurons containing twisted protein filaments. No one then could begin to fathom the significance of this matter.

In fact, researcher and geneticist Rudolf Tanzi observed that trying to comprehend what he saw was the equivalent of a person who had never seen a football game trying to understand the game by looking at the stands, the litter, and the dug-up dirt after the game was over. Even after possibly finding a torn page from a playbook, it would be impossible for such a person to understand the game of football (Gross, 2001).

Our understanding of this debilitating disease has continued to progress. By the late 1980s, scientists were beginning to isolate the protein that forms the plaque on the brain cells of individuals living with Alzheimer's. Researchers suddenly had a clearer picture of how neurons containing twisted protein filaments came to be. They began to understand how these tangles, as they are called, destroy brain cells—taking familiar names, faces, and places with them.

Researchers continue to discover multiple causes for the onset of the disease as they further their understanding of the relationship between the amyloid and tau proteins and identify the environmental factors that may play a part. Their work to date represents an extraordinary feat for biological research.

These discoveries mark one side of the coin in understanding Alzheimer's. The other side, which is equally significant, is the current movement toward attending to the psychosocial and humanistic aspects of dementia care.

Those of us in the field of dementia care are reexamining our philosophical beliefs and exploring practical, hands-on approaches in our relationships with individuals living with Alzheimer's disease. We are creating innovative programs and developing a new framework for preserving the emotional health, autonomy, and dignity of those who need us to walk hand in hand with them, witnessing the process of their experiences with empathy and respect.

Movement with Meaning™ is one such program. Designed for persons in the early stage of Alzheimer's disease, Movement with Meaning reinforces the remaining strengths and abilities of people with dementia by using a multisensory approach that stimulates all five senses. Practical and interactive by nature, the curriculum is ideal for physical therapists, recreational instructors, and activity directors in adult day centers and assisted living facilities, as well as health care professionals who are senior trainers and music or dance therapists.

Movement with Meaning provides an opportunity for each participant to become focused in the present through total immersion in short, concentrated exercises that stimulate physical, mental, and sensory awareness in a nurturing, contained environment.

When all channels—both sensory and intellectual—are open, an increase in self-awareness enables individuals with Alzheimer's disease to maintain their highest level of functioning. Each person is acknowledged and empowered by having the essence of his or her unique self affirmed. Movement with Meaning presents a new approach in exploring the personal and universal aspects of the mind of an individual with Alzheimer's disease. It is a program in which a person with Alzheimer's can investigate the landscape of his or her essential nature beyond the context of the disease.

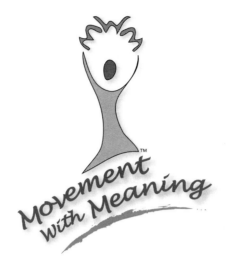

1

The Philosophy
of Movement with Meaning™

> "They carried the truth
> of themselves in a sheltered
> place inside the flesh, exactly the
> way a fruit that has gone soft still carries
> inside itself the clean hard stone of its future."

—Barbara Kingsolver (1989)

When we hear the word *Alzheimer's*, our initial reaction is often a chilling feeling followed by an equally charged sense of loss. Our imagination may conjure pictures of the brain being engulfed in a cool mist, lights slowly dimming, or other visions that represent an overwhelming sense of fading away. But it is important to understand that the loss of memory and cognitive functioning does not mean the loss of a person's uniqueness as a human being.

On the surface, the Alzheimer's mind seems like a deserted residence, but we can find folklore and legends to be rediscovered within its corridors. Many skills, feelings, and experiences are embodied within older adults with Alzheimer's disease because of the lives they've led. Each person represents a bounty of resources to be used in rediscovering the self. Whatever was lost in the cognitive realm can be recalled through the senses. For this reason, it is critical to separate the disease from the person (Woods, 1999). Yet, on another level, we must embrace the individual within the context of the disease to some degree. How the person with Alzheimer's disease is affected cannot be separated from his or her individual experience. Over the years, I have witnessed the tenacity and determination of the human spirit to express itself, finding any avenue to do so. This is the essence of Movement with Meaning™—to grab on to these innate experiences before the mist turns into fog, before the lights go out.

Why is it that a person with Alzheimer's disease cannot remember what he or she had for breakfast or the name of last night's movie but can vividly remember a poem from childhood or a song from the past? Perhaps the simplest way to explain this phenomenon is to examine the functions of the various parts of the brain.

Researchers have found that memory processes—taking in information, storing it, and retrieving it—are carried out by different parts of the brain. New memories are made and stored deep in a structure called the hippocampus. Individuals in early-stage Alzheimer's disease have damage to the hippocampus, which affects short-term memory. They do not, however, experience damage to the cerebral cortex, where long-term memory is stored (Rodgers, 2004). As a result, they can remember things from the distant past.

Because these long-term memories are preserved, the challenge is to assist the individual with Alzheimer's disease in retrieving them. Repetition is an effective tool to retrieve memories (Burns, McCarten, Adler, Bauer, & Kuskowski, 2004). In Movement with Meaning, the multisensory activities in each class are divided into five segments that create a choreography of movements in which short, repetitive exercises increase a sense of well-being. The repetition of activities enables the person with Alzheimer's disease not only to refamiliarize him- or herself with a specific poem, song, or hymn but also to embody the present.

One of the first subtle effects of Alzheimer's disease is disorientation. When a person with Alzheimer's disease becomes lost in familiar surroundings—not knowing where he or she is or how to get home—an increase in anxiety can occur. With this anxiety comes a sense of bewilderment and confusion. The underlying question becomes, "Where is my body in time and space?" It is therefore imperative that the word *home* take on a deeper meaning regarding disorientation. *Home* refers to the core of our essential being, the core of the body (Fazio, Seman, & Stansell, 1999).

In Movement with Meaning, the body becomes the container through which the person with Alzheimer's disease can feel empowered. This is why the classes begin with simple breathing techniques that are very effective for relaxing the mind and the body and for bringing the individual into the present moment. By using a mindful breathing practice to address the issues of disorientation in a person in early-stage Alzheimer's disease, it is possible to prevent the sense of feeling overwhelmed and replace it with the ability to focus with greater clarity and peace of mind.

Determining where one exists in physical space is the result of an ongoing interaction based on knowledge of both the starting point and the direction in which one has moved. To be able to comprehend where the body is in time and space—to be able to navigate the environment—is crucial for independence.

The yoga postures and bilateral integration exercises in Movement with Meaning stimulate both the right and left hemispheres of the brain. A sense of equilibrium is enhanced when the midline of the body is in alignment with the earth. Increasing spatial awareness enhances balance and coordination.

Early in the disease process, verbal communication skills become impaired. Individuals may have difficulty finding the right word or naming common objects. They might make errors in speech, such as saying "baffet" instead of "basket." Although these words have gone, familiar songs, prayers, hymns, and poems learned early in life are still rooted in long-term memory. These retained memories, developed throughout a lifetime, are part of the person. They are, in the case of a person with Alzheimer's disease, the basis of self-worth (Schmall, Cleland, & Sturdevant, 2000).

In Movement with Meaning, memorizing a short poem can cue reminiscence, bringing back images and feelings from the past. Incorporating percussion instruments, music, and dance into the multisensory activities reinforces confidence and increases visual, auditory, and kinesthetic awareness.

When the elements of Movement with Meaning are put together in a daily program, attention is refocused back on the body of the person with Alzheimer's disease. After all, many individuals are aware of the nature of their disease and the ways in which it is altering their lives.

Why wait until the disease progresses, watching the skills that are still intact slowly fade like a photograph that has been exposed to the sun too long? The time is now, in the early stage, to reinforce remaining strengths and abilities (Karp et al., 2004). The time is now, while the individual is aware of his or her personal biography, to investigate the sense of how the individual's inner landscape is changing. The time is now to create an environment that strives to preserve the identity and dignity of each individual affected by Alzheimer's disease.

Movement with Meaning is a program that focuses on connecting—on a very personal level—with each unique individual. Instead of defining people by their disease, the program presents a vital opportunity to open up new avenues for bonding. It is a journey through the senses, an excursion through the corridors of the mind where legends can be discovered.

2

Interviewing and
Selecting Participants

"I write so
often of people with no
magnitude, at least on the surface. I write of 'little people.' But are
there 'little people'? Sometimes I think
there are only little conceptions of people.
Whatever is living and feeling with intensity
is not little, and examined in depth, it would
seem to me that most 'little people' are living
with that intensity that I can use as a writer."

—Tennessee Williams (1972)

Every human being has a personal history, reflected time
and again in visible endowments and rooted in invisible
gifts that have been knitted into the fabric of everyday life.
Movement with Meaning™ offers individuals in early-stage
Alzheimer's disease a glimpse into this internal landscape.
The very nature of the short, repetitive activities and exercises assists the participant in experiencing the body as an
anchor to the present. By being embodied in the present
moment, an individual is free to cross the bridge between

the present and the past without fear of becoming confused or disoriented. The person can then explore and delve into the rich texture of the living, breathing past.

The life-enhancing potential for individuals who benefit from Movement with Meaning is multiple and diverse; however, the success of any program is based on effective screening criteria that can best meet the needs and interests of the participating individuals.

An ongoing issue in the field of Alzheimer's care is whether it is important for the individual with Alzheimer's disease to acknowledge that he or she has the disease. This is a personal and delicate issue (Kuhn, 1999). I have found that it is not necessary for individuals participating in Movement with Meaning to know the specifics of their diagnosis; it is a good idea, however, to explore knowledge of memory loss with them without being too intrusive.

It also is reassuring for some individuals to know that they have Alzheimer's disease. But for many, the process of accepting the diagnosis is a gradual one. Either way, it is important to consider that each person's temperament and personality is unique. It is essential that health care professionals remain aware at all times of the more subtle ways a person can communicate the experience of memory loss. One participant in a Movement with Meaning class stated, "My memory feels so elastic." This is a poignant metaphorical description of the core of her experience (Paige, 1999).

Instead of focusing on what is absent, Movement with Meaning revitalizes the sometimes dormant energies in the body and senses of the individual in early-stage Alzheimer's disease. Using what is present and functioning now gives an individual an appreciation of the skills and abilities that are still intact. It is therefore important for the staff in dementia care to see the person as a whole being. Knowing an individual's biography and what has brought him or her pleasure and passion frees the staff from having to superimpose an activity that may be boring or inappropriate.

Staff members have the opportunity to be fully aware of the personal history of potential participants attending adult day care programs or residing in assisted living facilities. They have an understanding of the psychological and emotional needs of the individuals in their charge. Movement with Meaning is easily incorporated into these settings, and therefore a formal screening may not be necessary.

Health care professionals who are physical therapists, senior trainers, or music and dance therapists may see an opportunity to implement a Movement with Meaning class within their private practices. I encourage them to do so, assuming that they have had personal experience working with individuals with Alzheimer's disease. It is essential that they feel comfortable with these individuals and have a desire to connect with them in a personal and spiritual way.

The key to a successful program is to ensure that a potential participant is suitable for Movement with Meaning. It is important to establish clear and concise guidelines to make an informed decision about who will benefit from the program (Yale, 1995). The following criteria will help professionals in adult day care programs, assisted living facilities, and private practices to select those individuals who will be appropriate for Movement with Meaning:

1. The individual has a diagnosis of early-stage Alzheimer's disease or a related disorder, such as Lewy Bodies disease, Pick's disease, vascular dementia, or Parkinson's disease with dementia.

2. The individual enjoys social activities that involve physical exercise.

3. The individual has basic communication skills and can understand simple directions.

4. The individual can participate in a Movement with Meaning class for 30 minutes, three to five times a week, without experiencing incontinence or showing combative or aggressive behaviors.

5. The individual is interested in participating in Movement with Meaning and willingly agrees to participate.

6. The individual is able to respond correctly in word and gestures to three of the five pretest exercises given in the Potential Participant Intake Questionnaire (see page 18).

7. The individual has a family caregiver or responsible person to contact.

These guidelines give health care professionals a context within which they can determine whether an individual in early-stage Alzheimer's disease may benefit from Movement with Meaning. Nothing, however, can replace the knowledge and understanding of each individual and his or her unique experience with the disease.

The building blocks for any trusting relationship are listening, affirming, and accepting. The health care professional must add an investigative component for trust to exist. It is important to be able to explore, wait, and find a thread of commonality between the health care professional and the individual with Alzheimer's disease (Bell & Troxel, 1997).

For health care professionals who have a private practice in dementia care, administering an initial caregiver questionnaire is necessary to become familiar with the potential participant's living situation. Family caregivers can provide important information on how they perceive their loved one's functional level, as well as how that person might do in a Movement with Meaning class.

If at all possible, conduct an in-home interview with both the caregiver and the potential participant. This sets a trusting atmosphere in which you can discuss the benefits of a Movement with Meaning class. I have found that if I state at the beginning of the interview that I would like to speak with each person individually during the screening process, the caregiver and his or her loved one are very willing to do so.

The process for selecting a participant for a Movement with Meaning class involves both practical and intuitive criteria. The Caregiver Intake Questionnaire (see page 12) will help you better assess how each individual may benefit from participating in a Movement with Meaning class. Taking the time to complete a thorough assessment will save you from repeated telephone calls or in-home visits. Also, you won't be placing the caregiver and his or her loved one in an awkward situation if the potential participant does not meet the criteria for a Movement with Meaning class. The following review of the Caregiver Intake Questionnaire will serve as a guide to help you better understand the underlying intent of each question:

Question 1: Seeking a professional evaluation of a loved one's impairment is essential. The term *dementia* refers to multiple symptoms that characterize certain diseases and conditions affecting intellectual functioning. In and of itself, *dementia* is a somewhat vague term unless the following question is asked: "Why are these symptoms being presented?" Symptoms usually associated with dementia can result from a variety of reversible conditions, such as urinary tract infection, nutritional imbalance, reactions to medications, and thyroid problems. But Alzheimer's disease and other related forms of dementia are irreversible forms of dementia. They require a careful, comprehensive evaluation that includes an account of the person's history, a physical examination, blood tests, neurological examinations, and brain scans, such as a magnetic resonance imaging (MRI), a single photon emission computed tomography (SPECT), a positron emission tomography (PET), and an electrocardiogram (EKG). A simple Folstein Mini-Mental Status Examination (Folstein, 2001) is a common tool used to determine if the symptoms of dementia are present, but it does not indicate whether the condition is irreversible or reversible (Shankle & Amen, 2004).

Questions 2 and 3: Although it is not important for the loved one to be aware of his or her diagnosis to participate in a

Caregiver
Intake Questionnaire

Person conducting interview: _____ Date: _____

Family member: _____

Potential participant: _____

Date of birth: _____ Age: _____ Gender: _____

Relationship of family member to potential participant: _____

Address: _____

Telephone: _____

How the person heard about Movement with Meaning™: _____

_____

1. Has your loved one had a comprehensive evaluation indicating a diagnosis of Alzheimer's disease or a related dementia such as Lewy Bodies disease, Pick's disease, vascular dementia, or Parkinson's disease with dementia?

    By whom:_____

    Date:_____

2. Is your loved one aware of the diagnosis?

3. Can your loved one discuss how he or she experiences and feels about the disease?

4. Does your loved one have difficulty with

    ☐ Remembering what day it is

    ☐ Sometimes getting lost

    ☐ Recalling names of friends or family members

    ☐ Writing or reading

    ☐ Finding the right word in a conversation

Source: Yale (1995). Adapted with permission.

From *Movement with Meaning: A Multisensory Program for Individuals with Early-Stage Alzheimer's Disease.* © 2006 Barbara Larsen. Published by Health Professions Press, Inc. (http://www.healthpropress.com). All rights reserved.

☐ Driving

☐ Managing money

☐ Coordination or balance

☐ Poor concentration

5. Is your loved one able to communicate his or her thoughts and understand simple directions?

6. Does your loved one enjoy small-group activities and social interactions?

7. Does your loved one have any physical limitations, such as

☐ Vision or hearing loss

☐ Difficulty with speech

☐ Mobility problems

☐ A recent surgery

☐ Other

8. Are you concerned about your loved one's moods? Does he or she show signs of anxiety, depression, delusions, or hallucinations?

9. Does your loved one have any current behavior problems, such as agitation, restlessness, or combativeness?

10. Can your loved one participate in a 30-minute class without bladder or bowel problems?

11. Do you think your loved one will be able to stay interested and focused in a Movement with Meaning class that meets three to five times a week?

12. Does your loved one have any other significant medical problems?

Source: Yale (1995). Adapted with permission.

From *Movement with Meaning: A Multisensory Program for Individuals with Early-Stage Alzheimer's Disease.* © 2006 Barbara Larsen. Published by Health Professions Press, Inc. (http://www.healthpropress.com). All rights reserved.

13. What medications, if any, is your loved one currently taking?

14. Does your loved one have any allergies that are flower- or plant-based (e.g., lavender, rose)?

15. What interests or hobbies does your loved one have now?

16. What was your loved one's career or occupation?

17. Earlier in life, what hobbies or social activities did your loved one enjoy?

18. Is there anything else you would like to discuss or share with me regarding Movement with Meaning or your loved one?

Source: Yale (1995). Adapted with permission.

From *Movement with Meaning: A Multisensory Program for Individuals with Early-Stage Alzheimer's Disease.* © 2006 Barbara Larsen. Published by Health Professions Press, Inc. (http://www.healthpropress.com). All rights reserved.

Movement with Meaning class, any sense of awareness of the condition can help lessen frustration when interacting in a group setting. The main focus is that the loved one enjoy and experience pleasure from being in the class.

Question 4: The symptoms associated with early-stage Alzheimer's disease provide a context, as well as guideposts, for understanding the disease. It is important to be aware, however, that the manifestation of these symptoms is individual in nature. Although one person may show a deficit in two or three symptoms, another individual may seem to manifest many of the symptoms simultaneously.

Question 5: Comprehending simple directions is critical and will be determined during the interview with the potential participant. The underlying question is, "Can your loved one follow a simple command?"

Question 6: This question is self-explanatory, but it is important to know if the loved one enjoys being with others in a social setting.

Question 7: Physical limitations may interfere with a participant's ability to receive the benefits of a Movement with Meaning class. How does the loved one's limitation(s) affect his or her functional level? Health care professionals who work with individuals in early-stage Alzheimer's disease who use a wheelchair for mobility should note that these individuals can still benefit from a Movement with Meaning class. This would involve some innovative and creative thinking, but for those professionals who work with individuals with physical disabilities, it may be a pleasant opportunity to try something new. The emphasis would be on expanding the bilateral exercises and yoga postures for the arms and upper body. In classes 2 and 4 in which a simple dance sequence is used, the participants can use their wheelchairs to form the circle and not be concerned about holding hands.

Questions 8 and 9: Behavior problems vary with each individual and usually do not occur until the middle stage of Alzheimer's disease. If there are any significant problems, however, it is imperative to ask the caregiver if this is a recent phenomenon and to determine what may have triggered the problem. The underlying question is whether the loved one's behavior would disrupt a Movement with Meaning class.

Question 10: If the person has a minor bladder problem, this can be dealt with by making sure that he or she uses the bathroom before class begins.

Question 11: This focuses on the basic temperament and personality of the loved one. Many people are not fond of a structured environment because it is not consistent with how they have lived their lives. Inquire if the loved one enjoys staying with an activity or project over a long period of time. Consistency is extremely important for a participant to reap the benefits of a Movement with Meaning class. The commitment to participate is essential and helps to foster a cohesive environment among the participants.

Question 12: Awareness of significant health problems gives you an idea of what to expect from each participant.

Question 13: It is important to be aware of any medications the person is taking and their possible side effects.

Question 14: This question is important because aromatherapy may be used in a Movement with Meaning class.

Questions 15, 16, and 17: These questions are designed to help you discover who the person is behind the mask of Alzheimer's disease. What are his or her gifts and talents? What gave him or her pleasure in the earlier years, and what abilities are still intact? These questions will help you find a thread of commonality from which to connect to the potential participant.

Question 18: This is an open-ended question that the caregiver may respond to in any way.

When the interview with the family caregiver has been completed, ask to meet with the potential participant. This is your private time together to explore and identify the potential participant's abilities, talents, and skills. But more important, this time is for you to investigate the characteristics that define this unique individual.

As with the Caregiver Intake Questionnaire, the Potential Participant Intake Questionnaire (see page 18) gives you an in-depth opportunity to determine whether the individual will benefit from a Movement with Meaning class.

Before beginning the Potential Participant Intake Questionnaire, take time to sit near the potential participant so you can maintain good eye contact with him or her. Speak slowly and clearly. It is crucial to establish a friendly, warm rapport with the potential participant. Before asking the first question, discuss why you are there, as noted in the introduction.

Question 1: Individuals in early-stage Alzheimer's disease have an incredible memory when it comes to their early childhood experiences. This question sets a friendly tone and helps you understand the values and traditions with which the individual with Alzheimer's disease was raised.

Questions 2 and 3: Occupation and interests help establish meaning and purpose in life. Many people were involved in their communities and churches. They belonged to clubs and volunteer organizations. These questions help give you a bigger picture of what was important to this person in his or her childhood and early adult years.

Question 4: Many hobbies and activities from the past are still important to the individual in early-stage Alzheimer's disease. He or she may enjoy playing golf, playing the piano, painting, fishing, collecting coins or stamps, and so forth. This question will help you integrate a participant's special interest with a theme from one of the Movement with Meaning classes.

Questions 5, 6, and 7: These may be delicate questions for the potential participant to answer. Let the individual gauge

Potential Participant
Intake Questionnaire

Person conducting interview: _____   Date: _____

Name of potential participant: _____

I am here today to see if you might be interested in joining a class to improve your memory, balance, and coordination through activities such as singing, memory games, dancing, and exercise. First, I would like to ask you a few questions.

1. Tell me some things about yourself.

    •   Where were you raised?

    •   What did your parents do for work?

    •   Do you come from a small or a large family?

    •   What is one thing that stands out in your mind when you think of your childhood?

2. What career or occupation were you involved with in your early years?

3. What hobbies or particular interests did you have in your early years?

4. What hobbies or activities do you enjoy now?

5. Please tell me if you have any difficulty with

    ☐ Remembering what day it is

    ☐ Sometimes getting lost

    ☐ Recalling names of friends or family members

    ☐ Writing or reading

    ☐ Finding the right word in a conversation

    ☐ Driving

    ☐ Managing your money

    ☐ Walking or balancing

Source: Yale (1995). Adapted with permission.

6. Please tell me the reason you think you have been experiencing difficulty with
_____.

7. Do these things concern you?

8. Do you think you would enjoy being in a class three to five times a week to improve your memory and balance through activities such as singing, memory games, dancing, and exercise to help you retain your special abilities and talents?

9. What questions do you have about the class?

Pretest Exercises

Now I would like to do some exercises with you. This will help me understand your strengths.

1. Ask the potential participant to walk to a specific place in the room and walk back to you.

2. Have the individual sit in a chair with his or her eyes closed. Ask the individual to tell you when he or she feels your finger on his or her left shoulder, right shoulder, left elbow, right elbow, left knee, and right knee.

3. Ask the potential participant to stand against a wall and raise his or her right arm above the head, then the left arm above the head. Ask the individual to raise up the right knee, then the left knee.

4. Ask the participant to finish these sentences.
   A dog wags his_____.
   A valentine box is full of_____.
   A squirrel climbs a_____.

5. Give the potential participant a piece of paper with either four letters or numbers written in large print (e.g., 5849, BFTC). Have the person look at the numbers for approximately 20 seconds. Read the letters or numbers once with him or her. Take away the paper and ask the potential participant to repeat the letters or numbers in sequence.

Thank you for taking the time to answer these questions and participate in the exercises. If you think of anything that you would like to discuss about this class, please feel free to contact me.

Source: Yale (1995). Adapted with permission.

From *Movement with Meaning: A Multisensory Program for Individuals with Early-Stage Alzheimer's Disease.* © 2006 Barbara Larsen. Published by Health Professions Press, Inc. (http://www.healthpropress.com). All rights reserved.

how comfortable he or she is with these questions. If you sense any frustration or embarrassment, move on to the next question.

Question 8: It is important for the potential participant to have a personal interest in joining a class. Enjoyment is the key for any program to be successful.

Question 9: This question is self-explanatory. Many individuals do not have questions at the end of the interview. I encourage potential participants to think about joining the class and to contact me if they think of any questions in the near future.

The second half of the interview will help you assess the physical and mental functional ability of the potential participant.

Activity 1: Can the individual follow simple directions? Although most of the exercises in a Movement with Meaning class are presented in a context of mirroring and repeating what the instructor is doing or saying, a participant who cannot follow simple directions is likely to become frustrated.

Activity 2: Does the individual have a sense of his or her body in time and space? You can assist the potential participant by first stating that you are going to place your finger on his or her left shoulder so as not to startle him or her.

Activity 3: Does the individual show any problems with range of motion, balance, or coordination? The wall will help support the potential participant. The height of the knee is not as important as the ability to balance with the assistance of a prop (wall or chair).

Activities 4 and 5: How does the individual fare with auditory and visual sequential memory? The multisensory activities in Movement with Meaning involve sequential memory skills. It is acceptable if the individual responds appropriately to two of three in Activity 4 and three of four letters or numbers in sequence in Activity 5.

For the potential participant to be able to fully benefit from a Movement with Meaning class, he or she should pass three of five exercises. However, pay attention to your intuition and personal experience with each individual to make this determination. There are no strict rules—only guidelines to help you address this issue.

SAMPLE OBSERVATION SHEET

New horizons in early-stage Alzheimer's care are beginning to emerge. Yet this is still a relatively new field. Advocacy is invaluable. Education and documentation help to increase the visibility of innovative programs. Careful documentation may provide the necessary data for policy makers, private institutions, and research centers to support new programs through grant funding (Yale, 1995).

The sample Observation of Participant Form (see page 22) charts the level of participation of each individual on a weekly basis. You are encouraged, however, to make daily informal notations to yourself in a nonintrusive manner at the end of each class.

A Movement with Meaning class is composed of five segments with an overall theme to reinforce continuity, concentration, and awareness. The charting has been categorized by number, indicating whether there has been "no change" in the participant's experience of an activity or exercise, "slight improvement," "moderate improvement," or finally, "significant improvement." This type of charting may at first seem vague, but as you feel more comfortable with the natural rhythm and choreography of a Movement with Meaning class, your awareness will focus on the subtle aspects of how each participant is progressing.

Record your impressions informally until you have completed a couple of weeks of a Movement with Meaning class. Once you begin to know the participants on a more intimate level, you will be able to document your observations. The Comments section at the end of the form is

Observation of Participant Form

Name:_____

Date: _____ Class number: _____

For each participant, chart any changes in participation in the numbered categories listed below. This change should be noted at the end of each week:
1 = no change; **2** = slight improvement; **3** = moderate improvement;
4 = significant improvement.

Participation in Segment 1: Centering through breathing

Ability to focus: _____

Participation in Segment 2: Memorization/visualization

Ability to concentrate: _____

Verbal expression: _____

Participation in Segment 3: Bilateral integration exercises/yoga

Coordination and
balance: _____

Ability to anticipate
sequence: _____

Participation in Segment 4: Music, rhythm, and movement

Ability to coordinate poem
or song with percussion
instrument: _____

Ability to coordinate poem
or song with dance
steps: _____

Ability to anticipate
sequence: _____

Participation in Segment 5: Sensory stimulation

Verbal expression: _____

Expression of emotion: _____

Comments:

provided for users to describe the nonverbal behaviors of the participants. Communication can be very subtle through facial expressions and body language. If a specific issue arises regarding how the participant interacts with the other members of the class, you can elaborate on that in this section. It is important to record anything that may further your understanding of what each participant experiences in a Movement with Meaning class.

PROMOTING PUBLIC RELATIONS AND COMMUNITY AWARENESS

Since the start of the 21st century, early detection methods in Alzheimer's disease research have continued to improve. Concerns are mounting regarding treatment options that constructively assist people with Alzheimer's disease to retain and nurture what makes them uniquely human. As the general public becomes more educated about the needs of their loved ones in the early stage of Alzheimer's disease, expectations for reshaping and implementing new ways of caring will challenge existing programs.

Promoting any new program may seem overwhelming at first. Beginning at the grassroots level is an easy and comfortable way to help the public and health care professionals understand the positive effects of a Movement with Meaning class. Consider the following avenues for recruiting potential participants:

- Ask to speak at your local caregiver support group(s) or a support group for individuals with early-stage Alzheimer's disease.

- Request an interview on a community radio program about health or senior issues.

- Write an article for a newspaper as an educational piece for community awareness.

- Meet with staff of health care agencies or facilities (e.g., home care, adult day care centers, assisted living facilities, research centers, hospital social workers, discharge planners).

- Network with local, state, and county employees who work in the field of elder care.

- Create a flier (see Figure 2.1) for an introductory workshop on Movement with Meaning.

Your community may have an elder care providers' coalition or council where health care professionals meet on a monthly basis. It may take time to find the resources in your community, but the awareness of the general public is ever-evolving. As the baby boomers become "elder boomers," a new generation is emerging, and these individuals are not afraid to rebel against the status quo mentality regarding health care.

SAMPLE RELEASE AND WAIVER OF LIABILITY FORM

Any program involving physical exercise has a risk of injury. Ensuring the safety of each participant in a Movement with Meaning class requires careful screening to prevent any serious physical injury. As the instructor, you must be aware and vigilant—intuitively as well as cognitively. For the staff of adult day care centers and assisted living facilities, a Release and Waiver of Liability form (see page 27) would normally be signed by the participant or resident and caregiver at the time of the application and intake process. For private instructors who are in the field of dementia care, a waiver form is imperative to acknowledge the limits of professional responsibility (Yale, 1995). This ensures a clear understanding on the part of the participant and his or her caregiver that they are freely consenting to participate in a Movement with Meaning class by signing the release of liability form.

MOVEMENT WITH MEANING™

A multisensory program for individuals with early-stage Alzheimer's disease or related dementia

Presented by
Barbara Larsen, M.A. Ed.

Saturday, June 24, 2005
9:00 a.m. to 11:00 a.m.
Main Street Yoga Center
100 Main Street
Nevada City

Family caregivers and individuals with early-stage Alzheimer's disease or related dementia are invited to attend a FREE introductory workshop for potential participants to enhance concentration, body posture, spatial awareness, and memory through:

Breathing and centering techniques

Memorization and visualization activities

Yoga and bilateral integration exercises

Music, rhythm, and movement activities

Multisensory awareness techniques

For further information or to register, call [telephone number]

Figure 2.1. Sample flier to promote participation in the Movement with Meaning program. This sample announces a free introductory class.

Once thoughtful consideration has been given to laying the groundwork for a Movement with Meaning class, the fun begins. Knowing who your participants are as unique individuals—with your focus on the person as a whole being—allows you the opportunity to relax and feel confident as you witness their journeys with Alzheimer's disease.

You become a conduit, providing a glimpse into their unique internal landscapes through a multisensory approach that explores their rich histories while anchoring them to the present.

MOVEMENT WITH MEANING™
Release and Waiver of Liability

Because physical exercise can be subject to risk of injury, you are urged to obtain a physical examination from your physician before participating in a Movement with Meaning class. You agree that by participating in a Movement with Meaning class, you do so entirely at your own risk. You agree that you are voluntarily participating in the activities and exercises in this class and assume all risks of injury.

You acknowledge that you have carefully read this release and waiver of liability and fully understand that you expressly agree to release and discharge the instructor or the creator and author of Movement with Meaning, Barbara Larsen, from any and all claims or causes of action, and you agree to voluntarily give up or waive any right that you may otherwise have to bring legal action against the instructor or the creator and author of Movement with Meaning, Barbara Larsen, for personal injury.

To the extent that statute or case law does not prohibit releases for negligence, the release is also for negligence.

If any portion of this release and waiver of liability shall be deemed by a court of competent jurisdiction to be invalid, then the remainder of this release and waiver of liability shall remain in full force and effect and the offending provision or provisions severed herefrom.

By signing this release, I acknowledge that I understand its content and that this release and waiver of liability cannot be modified orally.

Name of participant: _____
(print name)

Signature of participant: _____

Address: _____

City, State, ZIP: _____

Telephone: _____Date:____/____/____

I, being the legal conservator or appointed legal attorney-in-fact through a Durable Power of Attorney of the named above, hereby consent to and join in the foregoing release and waiver of liability on behalf of said person.

Signed: _____Date:____/____/____

3

Setting the Environment

"And the place, never neutral
of course, will cast its influence."

—Frances Mayes (1996)

Individuals in early-stage Alzheimer's disease are very sensitive to their physical environment. Supportive and comfortable surroundings are essential, but the creation of a peaceful place that focuses on balancing individuals' internal and external realities is equally important (Fazio et al., 1999).

People with Alzheimer's disease hesitate when they are in a new situation or environment, and it is easy for them to become disoriented and confused (Alzheimer's Association, 1992). The optimal setting provides an atmosphere in which distant memories of songs, poems, and prayers can be retrieved and revisited in the here and now, connecting with each participant in a responsive and compassionate way.

CREATING A NURTURING ENVIRONMENT

It is critical to acknowledge and create a sense of sacred space for individuals with Alzheimer's. I use the word *sacred* to emphasize the care it takes to create an environment that fosters encouragement and successful experiences for each participant. Creating sacred space is about creating an environment filled with energy that comforts, supports, and uplifts. Sacred space can be created in any room or location, although designing the best setting for a Movement with Meaning™ class may take some planning and organizing. Consideration must be given to the multisensory exercises and activities as a whole. The dining room in an assisted living facility, for example, can be transformed into a cozy, comfortable environment (see Figure 3.1). The goal is for each participant to feel comfortable and safe in an environment that encourages independence and autonomy (Brawley, 1997; see Figure 3.2). When a quiet and nurturing environment is established, each participant can concentrate on being in the present, giving his or her authentic self the freedom to emerge.

DESIGNING A "SACRED SPACE"

The following recommendations will help create a successful sacred space:

- *Select a quiet location.* Find a room that is free from stimuli and distractions. Some participants become easily disoriented and agitated by voices or sounds in the background. Participants should not be near windows or doors with glass because their attention may be diverted by their reflections or outside activities.

- *Use the same room for each class.* Consistency is important for people with Alzheimer's disease. Predictability provides them with a sense of safety and empowerment.

- *Balance the seating arrangement.* Use sturdy chairs for comfort and safety. Allow space between the chairs for the movement exercises. Arrange the chairs in an oval or semicircle, facing you for good eye contact.

- *Optimize the size of the group.* Small groups of between six and eight participants work best to foster a sense of well-being. Each participant's abilities can be recognized and valued when there is a feeling of cohesiveness within the group.

- *Use props and materials.* Prepare for each class by having the equipment nearby. Make sure the audiotape is cued before each class. Check each percussion instrument. Handouts should be written in large print.

Creating the mood or ambiance for the class is a subtle process that involves using your intuitive nature. Does the room feel warm and inviting when a participant comes to class? Does it embody a trusting atmosphere? Is there a sense of being cared for? Consider the following suggestions when creating both a cheerful and sacred space:

- *Color and lighting create a mood.* Make sure that the colors in the room are soft and not busy. The lighting should be bright enough for the participants to see you and the props clearly but not too visually overwhelming to create an uncomfortable feeling.

- *Scents and fragrances heighten memories.* Some classes in Movement with Meaning incorporate the use of flowers and aromatherapy to reinforce a particular theme.

- *Music relieves tension and anxiety.* Select music with a slow tempo and a soft dynamic level. Classical and environmental music have a calming effect.

Creating a supportive, peaceful environment not only provides a safe haven from the everyday distractions that bombard the person with Alzheimer's disease, it also assures a predictable landmark that reinforces the routine and consistency of a Movement with Meaning class (Albrecht, 2003). By setting aside a specific place for Movement with Meaning, you are affirming your intention to enrich and deepen your connection with each participant. Sacred space becomes the container in which each participant can preserve and enhance his or her unique skills and abilities.

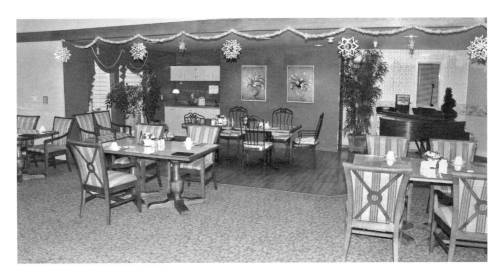

Figure 3.1. This dining room in an assisted living facility can be transformed into a cozy, comfortable environment (see next page).

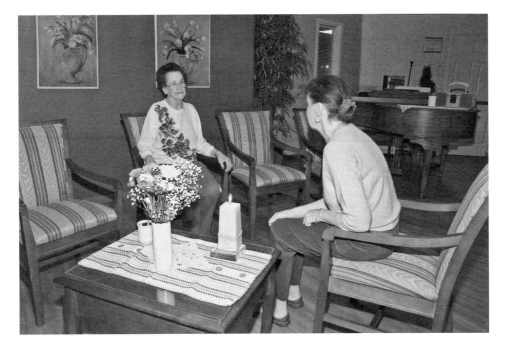

Figure 3.2. Each participant needs to feel comfortable and safe in an environment that encourages independence and autonomy.

4

Centering Through Breathing

"Breathing is the bridge to the mind."

—Donna Farhi (1996)

Individuals in early-stage Alzheimer's disease begin to experience difficulty remembering people's names, finding the right word, and orienting to time and place (Kuhn, 1999). This can be unsettling and cause fear and anxiety. Worrying about forgetting takes a lot of energy and contributes to a lack of concentration and attention. The mind becomes preoccupied with trying to understand what was just said or recognizing a familiar face. Ambiguity and confusion seem to be chronic states of being, and they become more apparent every day.

An excellent antidote to help diminish this anxiety and fear is mindful breathing, which serves as an anchor for the body and helps lift the mist of uncertainty that engulfs the mind (Higbee, 1996). Once the mind is calm and relaxed, concentration will follow, encouraging the body and one's essential self to connect. By connecting his or her internal landscape and the environment, the person with Alzheimer's disease may experience a subtle shift in awareness. What seems to occur is a willingness to inhabit one's body. The quality of being in the body is measured by a heightened sense of self (Suhr, Anderson, & Tranel, 1999). An individual is brought into the present moment through mindful breathing (Coulter, 2001).

Because mindful breathing sets the stage for a Movement with Meaning™ class, it is especially important to make sure that you, as the group leader, are relaxed and focused. You are the conduit for the activities in a Movement with Meaning class. The tone and mood that you create are interwoven with the multisensory exercises. It is your responsibility to be attentive, supportive, and energetic. Your mood is contagious, so you want it to be warm and friendly (Schmall et al., 2000). Before class, take a few minutes to connect with your breath. Follow the rhythm of breathing in and out. Visualize yourself strolling through a grassy meadow, watching the ocean waves as they ebb and flow, or relaxing in a personally peaceful setting.

Each Movement with Meaning class begins with mindful breathing. Chapter 10 illustrates four examples of Movement with Meaning classes that demonstrate how the rhythm and flow of each segment works with the theme. In this chapter, we focus on the first segment of the class: breathing exercises that reinforce relaxation and concentration.

Many of our older adults have never experienced mindful breathing. To sit quietly and focus inwardly may seem foreign or threatening; however, the participants seldom resist once they understand that the techniques enhance their memory or concentration.

Each breathing exercise is an attempt to explore and investigate the inner corridors of the mind. When a peaceful inner state has been established, the ability to retrieve firmly rooted songs, prayers, and poems can begin to resurface. The setting for the Movement with Meaning class has been established when each participant understands that this is "our sacred space."

SEGMENT 1

MINDFUL BREATHING

Make sure that you are familiar with each mindful breathing technique before you present it. Practice each exercise until you feel comfortable. Seating is arranged in a semicircle, with your chair in front of the participants (see Figure 4.1). After introductions, discuss the benefits of mindful breathing:

1. Mindful breathing helps us think more clearly.

2. Mindful breathing helps us remember.

3. Mindful breathing helps us feel stable in our bodies.

Begin by practicing each breathing exercise to get an idea of who may need direction with placement of feet, back, or hands (see Figure 4.2). Participants' feet should point straight ahead, a few inches apart; their backs should be straight, slightly touching the back of the chair; and their hands should be placed comfortably in their laps. As with all of the exercises and activities in any Movement with Meaning class, always compliment and reassure each participant in a respectful manner.

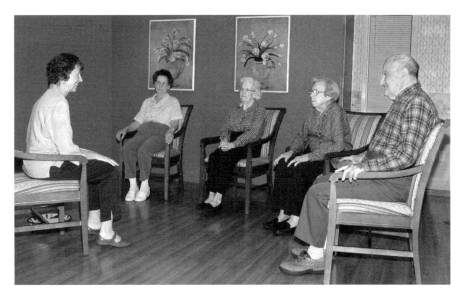

Figure 4.1. Arrange the seating for the mindful breathing exercises in a semicircle, with your chair in front of the participants.

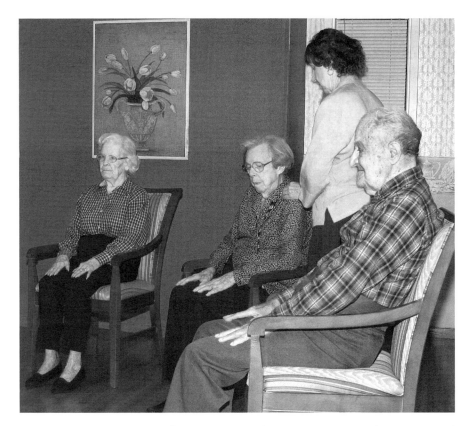

Figure 4.2. Practice each exercise so that you can see who may need direction with placement of his or her feet, back, or hands.

Mindful Breathing Exercise 1

Breathing Awareness

- Sit comfortably with your back straight and your feet pointing straight ahead.

- Close your eyes.

- Breathe normally, paying attention to each inhalation and exhalation.

- Begin to focus on the rhythm of your breathing.

- Silently count at the end of each out breath.

- Breathe in, breathe out—count "one."

- Breathe in, breathe out—count "two."

- Continue to count in this way up to 10.

- Repeat once.

For the first in and out breaths, count in a soft, clear voice. At the same time, remind participants to follow their own natural breathing rhythms.

Mindful Breathing Exercise 2
This–Now

- Sit comfortably with your back straight and your feet pointing straight ahead (see Figure 4.3).
- Close your eyes.
- Breathe normally, paying attention to each inhalation and exhalation.
- Repeat five times.
- Begin with an inhale, saying "this" to yourself.
- Exhale, saying "now" to yourself.
- Repeat 10 times, slowly.

It may be helpful to softly say, "inhale," "exhale," "this," and "now" until each participant feels comfortable with the technique.

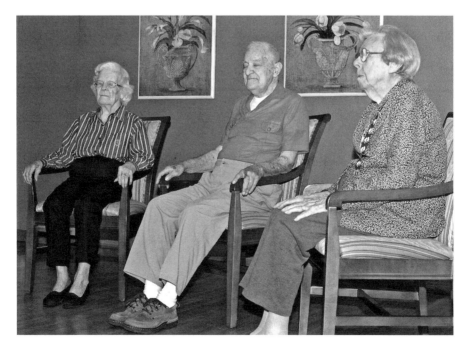

Figure 4.3. The participants demonstrate sitting comfortably with feet pointing straight ahead. They prepare to inhale by saying "this" and to exhale by saying "now."

Mindful Breathing Exercise 3

Conscious Breathing

> "Breathing in, I know I am
> breathing in.
> Breathing out, I know I am
> breathing out."
> —Thich Nhat Hanh (1991)

- Sit comfortably with your back straight and your feet pointing straight ahead.

- Close your eyes.

- Breathe normally, paying attention to each inhalation and exhalation.

- Repeat five times.

- Breathe in and say to yourself, "Breathing in, I know I am breathing in."

- Breathe out and say to yourself, "Breathing out, I know I am breathing out."

- Repeat 10 times.

Mindful Breathing Exercise 4

Soft Breathing

- Sit comfortably with your back straight and your feet pointing straight ahead.

- Close your eyes.

- Breathe normally, paying attention to each inhalation and exhalation.

- Repeat five times.

- Take a deep breath and repeat to yourself, "soft belly" (see Figure 4.4).

- Exhale and relax.

- Repeat 10 times.

- Breathe normally again.

As you practice these breathing techniques with your group, a sense of familiarity will help ensure trust, and the barriers of confusion and anxiety will lift. Each mindful breathing exercise has a rhythm that is recognizable in a way that feels safe because each participant can experience the connection between the mind and the body. Expressing her experience with mindful breathing, one participant stated, "I have enough to hold on to." This is the gift of awareness.

A teacher once told me, "Awareness does not come and go; we come and go with our attention." In other words, you "grow" your awareness by practicing mindful breathing.

The more we begin to understand what life must be like for individuals with Alzheimer's disease, the better we can appreciate how important and essential it is to create safe havens that allow them the potential to explore, express, and embrace their uniqueness as fellow travelers in this journey called life (Coste, 2003).

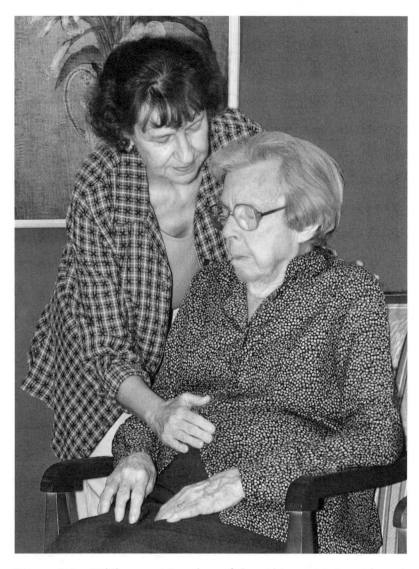

Figure 4.4. While practicing the soft breathing exercise, ask each participant to focus on relaxing the stomach muscles.

5

Learning by Heart

*"This man who was my
grandfather is present in me, as I
felt always his father to be present in him."*

—Wendell Berry (1992)

Human beings have both a personal and a collective history. The bridge between the past and the present is never traveled one way. We cannot possibly know who we are if we don't know where we have been. We carry not only the physical traits of our parents and ancestors but also their bloodlines. This gives us a sense of life as a continuum—a quality that seems everlasting (Campbell, 1988). As human beings, we need to embody our life stories. As neurologist Oliver Sacks stated, "We must 'recollect' ourselves, recollect the inner drama, the narrative, of ourselves. A man needs such a narrative, a continuous inner narrative, to maintain his identity, his self" (1985, p. 111).

Many older adults who were raised in the 1920s and 1930s were brought up with a deep connection to their past through long-standing family rituals. There was a rhythm to life, whether on the farm or in the city. Children knew their grandparents, aunts, uncles, and cousins. The extended family provided support, wisdom, and encouragement.

Family values, passed on by direct interaction between children and their relatives, gave order, meaning, and purpose to the family as a whole and to each individual member (Kotre, 1999–2000). Family gatherings during the holidays or festivals reinforced the significance of tradition and community and represented a strong sense of continuity. If children were in school, they were expected to memorize songs and poems. It was common to say, "I know it by heart" when referring to a prayer, song, or poem.

Individuals in early-stage Alzheimer's disease have a sense that there is "something not quite right" or "something the matter." As one participant put it, "I no longer feel like myself." Movement with Meaning™ creates a bridge between the past and present by revitalizing the sometimes dormant personal history of each participant.

The second segment of a Movement with Meaning class is memorizing a poem or song. Someone once said, "The muse of poetry is the muse of memory." Poems and songs that were learned early in life are stored in the long-term memory of the person with Alzheimer's disease and remain accessible to him or her (Kirkland & McIlveen, 1999). Recovering cherished poems and songs is important because it enhances the self-esteem and identity of the individual with Alzheimer's disease.

Repetition is the method for retrieving familiar poems and songs from the past, as well as for learning new poems and songs (Higbee, 1996). Expressing the rhythm pattern in poems and songs creates an atmosphere that is safe and nonthreatening and brings something to the lives of the participants that is representative of what was there before Alzheimer's disease.

Participants in a Movement with Meaning class are encouraged to bring poems or songs from their childhood and early adult years. One gentleman remembered the prologue to Chaucer's (1894) *Canterbury Tales*. He recited the first four lines from memory:

"Whan that Aprill with his shoures soote
The droghte of March hath perced to the roote,
And bathed every veyne in swich licour
Of which vertu engendred is the flour"
("When April with his showers sweet with fruit
The drought of March has pierced to the root,
And bathed each vein with liquor that has power
To generate therein and sire the flower")

We were all very impressed by his clear and passionate recitation. He shared with the class that he and his freshman classmates in college had to memorize the entire prologue. For a while his sense of time was erased, and the images of the short four-line prologue came flowing out effortlessly with his description of a spring day as his awakening brought him to the present moment. He was able to connect the past with the present in a very concrete way by using Chaucer's prologue as a frame of reference. It was also a very personal experience that validated his ability to retrieve a long, but not forgotten, poem.

In a way, this experience is metaphorical. Metaphor is how the body and the psyche talk to the conscious mind. These images can be expressed in both universal and personal terms. It is common for individuals with Alzheimer's disease to speak metaphorically (Bayley, 1999). When ordinary language expression seems to be locked within the plaques and tangles of the mind, every so often an experience can be expressed through the use of symbolic or metaphorical language.

While discussing how her aunt was adjusting to her new living situation, a caregiver recounted the following interaction with her relative. As the two women walked to the caregiver's car, the caregiver's aunt grabbed her arm and said, "If I didn't get to see you, it would be like soggy cigarette butts." Before getting into her car, the caregiver looked down and saw discarded cigarette butts in the gutter.

What a vivid imagination the aunt had in expressing her feelings so clearly in metaphorical terms!

The use of visualization techniques to expand on the images evoked by a poem or song is included in the second segment of a Movement with Meaning class. Visualization increases concentration because it creates focus on the more subtle "mental pictures" and "feelings" of a poem or song (Higbee, 1996). Together, memorization and visualization are the ideal ingredients for honoring both the past and the present.

SEGMENT 2

MEMORIZING A POEM OR SONG

After the mindful breathing exercise, introduce the poem or song for the next segment. You can write the poem or song on large index cards, making sure the writing is legible and in large print. Read the entire poem or song to the class for the first time. For the second reading, have everyone read the poem or song together (see Figure 5.1). You may want to do this several times until you feel that everyone is comfortable with the exercise before gathering up the cards. Then recite the poem or song line by line, asking the participants to repeat each line (see Figure 5.2). When the first line or phrase is memorized, move to the next line or phrase until the poem or song is memorized in its entirety.

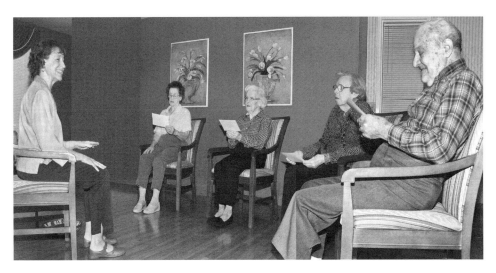

Figure 5.1.   Everyone in the group reads the poem or song together.

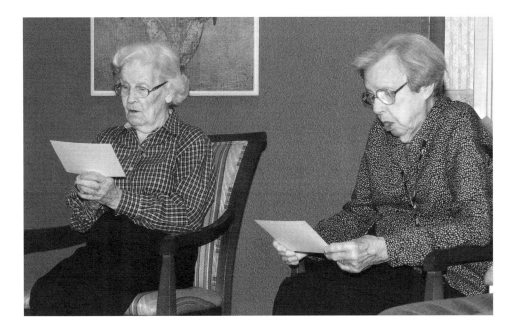

Figure 5.2.   Recite the poem or song line by line, asking the participants to repeat each line. When the first line or phrase is memorized, move to the next line or phrase.

Memorization Exercise 1

Poem: "The Pedigree of Honey"

"The pedigree of honey
Does not concern the bee;
A clover, any time, to him
Is aristocracy."
—Emily Dickinson (Todd & Higginson, 1982)

When all participants know the poem by heart, recite it one more time. Ask the participants to close their eyes. Then slowly read the poem (see Figure 5.3). This time, request that each participant be aware of any colors, shapes, feelings, or memories that may arise. After they open their eyes, ask if anyone would like to share his or her experience in a few words (see Figure 5.4).

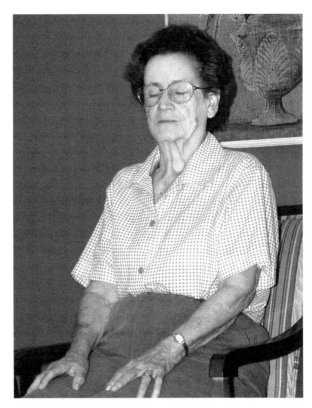

Figure 5.3. During the visualization exercise, ask the class members to close their eyes while you slowly recite the poem.

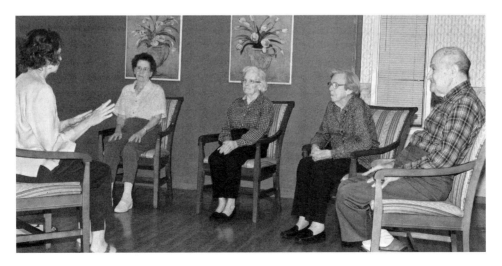

Figure 5.4. Allow time for the class members to share their experiences during the visualization exercise.

Memorization Exercise 2

Song: "Simple Gifts"

> "'Tis a gift to be simple, 'tis a gift to be free,
> 'Tis a gift to come down where we ought to be,
> And when we find ourselves in the place just right,
> 'Twill be in the valley of love and delight."
> —"Simple Gifts" (Fox, 1987)

A few of the participants may remember this song. You can find many songbooks in the library and in bookstores that have favorite American songs. This particular song was chosen because, just like its title, the words and melody are easy to remember. Sing the song in its entirety before asking the participants to repeat the song line by line. When the song is completely memorized, sing it together a few more times.

Ask the participants to close their eyes while you slowly sing the song. Ask them to pay attention to the last line, "'Twill be in the valley of love and delight." What images can they visualize (see Figure 5.5)? Sing the song once more, and ask the participants to recapture any images the song evokes for them (e.g., a warm, sunny day; grassy fields; birds flying). How does the song make them feel? Have them describe in a few words any memories this song may evoke (see Figure 5.6).

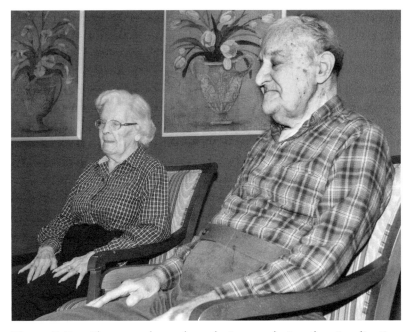

Figure 5.5.   Class members close their eyes during the visualization exercise while listening to the last line of "Simple Gifts."

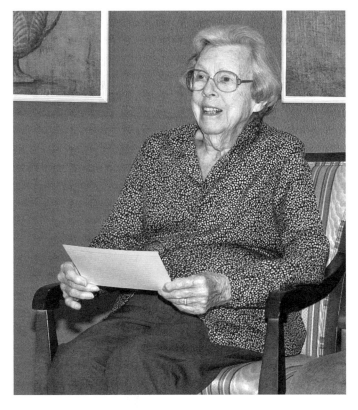

Figure 5.6.   Participant describes memories evoked by "Simple Gifts."

Memorization Exercise 3

Poem: "A Grain of Sand and a Wild Flower"

"To see a World in a Grain of Sand
And a Heaven in a Wild Flower,
Hold Infinity in the palm of your hand
And Eternity in an hour."
—William Blake (Kazin, 1968)

This poem by English poet William Blake is not easily understood, but the images in each line are very vivid and powerful. After memorizing this poem, one participant expressed, "I know there is more of me than here." She was able to sense a quality of timelessness in the poem.

Before you ask the participants to close their eyes while you recite the poem, reread key words and phrases from the poem: "grain of sand," "wild flower," "palm of your hand," and "eternity in an hour." Ask the participants to visualize these words and phrases. After they open their eyes, ask what colors, textures, feelings, and memories came to mind.

Song: "Sweet Betsy from Pike"

"Oh, don't you remember Sweet Betsy from Pike?
Who crossed the big mountains with her lover Ike.
With two yoke of oxen, a big yaller dog,
A tall Shanghai rooster, and one spotted hog."
—"Sweet Betsy from Pike" (Fox, 1987)

This favorite American folk song was popular during the Gold Rush in the middle of the nineteenth century. The tempo is lively and fun-spirited. Although participants sing only the first four lines of the song, the message is one of encouragement and hope.

Traditional folk songs and ballads are filled with allegory and potent memories. When singing a song, try to slow the tempo to grasp all of the rich images. Once again, ask the participants to close their eyes while you slowly sing the song, requesting that they be aware of the images. Which season is it? Are Betsy and Ike old or young? What color is the Shanghai rooster? Ask anyone if they would like to share, in a few words, memories that this song evokes.

In some respects, many individuals with Alzheimer's disease feel that the past has outmeasured the present's value. Movement with Meaning provides an environment in which distant memories of songs, poems, and hymns not only can be retrieved but also can serve as a refuge to be revisited time and again. Every time the bridge between the past and present is crossed, each participant is given the opportunity to investigate the treasures he or she has embodied from the past that can enrich the present and make it more sacred.

6

A Delicate Balance

*"Movement never lies.
It is a barometer telling the
state of the soul's weather."*

—Martha Graham (1991)

Movement is essential to human nature. People are designed to move. Spatial awareness is fundamental to understanding time and space as individuals respond to their surrounding world. To be aware of time and space requires one to be able to estimate the meaningful context within his or her environment. Individuals in early-stage Alzheimer's disease experience spatial disorientation because their physical and somatic cues are less intact, making it difficult to determine the position of their bodies in time and space.

Difficulties with spatial orientation affect motor ability. Although the motor cortex is in both hemispheres of the brain, the ability to make judgments based on the relationship of our bodies to space is centered in the right hemisphere.

Problems with balance and coordination begin to occur in early-stage Alzheimer's disease (Pettersson, Engardt, & Wahlund, 2002). There seems to be a loss of trust in the body, which is often exhibited by cautious movements. Individuals may hesitate, for example, when walking out the front door of the house, unsure whether to turn right or left to find the car.

To increase balance and coordination, Movement with Meaning™ works with bilateral integration exercises that enable people with Alzheimer's disease to feel safe and at *home* in their bodies. By aligning the body with the earth, a nonverbal statement is made: "I know where my body is in time and space."

Muscles love rhythmic movement. By satiating the body with repetitive bilateral movements, participants are not only integrating both left and right hemispheres of the brain but are also increasing their spatial awareness and finding refuge in the body (Drabben-Thiemann et al., 2002).

Each hemisphere of the brain specializes in certain skills and thinking characteristics. The left hemisphere is associated with reading, listening, following directions, learning language, identifying symbols, applying logic, and using sequential memory. The right hemisphere of the brain is associated with singing, playing music, visualizing, expressing emotions, understanding spatial relationships, and using intuition (Small, 2002). The bilateral integration exercises in Movement with Meaning focus on helping the participant identify the body's midline—the median plane where the left and right sides of the brain and body cross or overlap. Finding the center of one's body has not so much to do with the precision of body placement but rather with the more critical awareness of spatial orientation (Dennison & Dennison, 1994).

The bilateral exercises begin the third segment in the sequence of a Movement with Meaning class. These exercises can be alternated with the yoga postures in Chapter 7. By incorporating a physical component in a Movement with Meaning class, the transition from the cadence of a poem or the melody of a song is experienced as part of a continuum, unfolding a choreography of movements with a theme and purpose. The centering techniques, combined with poetry, music, and movement, help to contain and bring together the sometimes fragmented and disassociated self of the individual in early-stage Alzheimer's disease. Within this feeling of chaos is the essential, authentic self waiting to emerge and be recognized. The bilateral exercises and yoga postures are tools to assist the participants in becoming more alert and aware of their unique personhood.

To keep the flow of the movements in a meaningful context, I suggest that you use the same set of bilateral exercises for a class until you begin a new series, thereby creating a coherent and smooth transition from one segment to the next.

SEGMENT 3A

BILATERAL INTEGRATION EXERCISES

Discuss the benefits of bilateral exercises to maintain balance and coordination (Berg & Kairy, 2003). Demonstrate the first exercise as a way to introduce and explain the visual and kinesthetic value of these exercises. Make sure that there is enough space between chairs to allow for full movement of arms and legs. Arrange your chair so that each participant has clear eye contact with you. To ensure that the participants will be able to follow your instructions regarding which arm or leg to use, demonstrate that you are the mirror image of what they are doing. This saves a lot of time and unnecessary refocusing.

Bilateral Exercises 1a: Seated

Shoulder Shrugs

- Sit with your back straight and arms at your sides.
- Breathe normally.
- Lift your shoulders up toward your ears (see Figure 6.1).
- Lower your shoulders, relaxing your neck.
- Repeat five times.

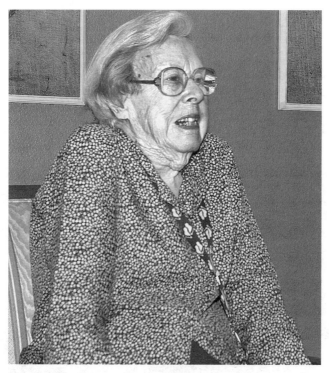

Figure 6.1. A participant lifts her shoulders up to her ears in the Shoulder Shrugs exercise.

Large Arm Circles

- Sit with your back straight and feet pointed straight ahead.

- Breathe normally.

- Keep your right arm straight as you circle your arm clockwise in front of your body (see Figure 6.2).

- Repeat three times.

- Circle your right arm counterclockwise.

- Repeat three times.

- Keep your left arm straight as you circle your arm clockwise in front of your body.

- Repeat three times.

- Circle your left arm counterclockwise.

- Repeat three times.

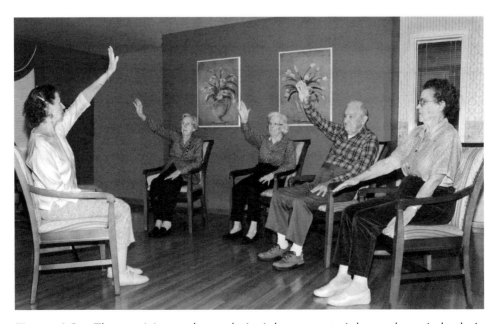

Figure 6.2. The participants keep their right arms straight as they circle their arms clockwise in front of their bodies.

Elbow Stretch and Cross

- Sit with your back straight and arms at your sides.

- Clasp your hands behind your neck with your elbows out to the side (see Figure 6.3).

- Exhale and bring your right elbow toward your left knee (see Figure 6.4).

- Keep your head straight while gazing at your left elbow.

- Inhale and straighten your torso (see Figure 6.5).

- Exhale and bring your left elbow toward your right knee.

- Keep your head straight while gazing at your right elbow.

- Inhale and straighten your torso.

- Repeat five times.

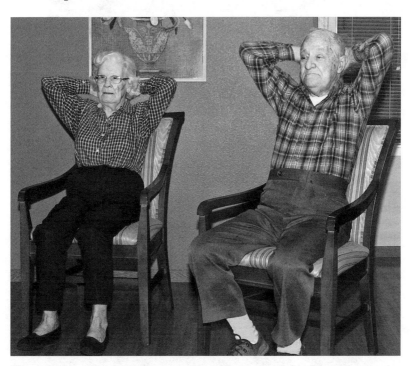

Figure 6.3. These class members take one of the first steps in the Elbow Stretch and Cross exercise.

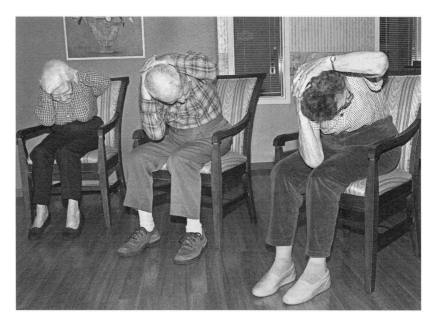

Figure 6.4. These participants bring their right elbows to their left knees.

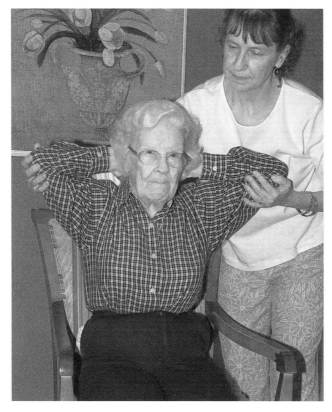

Figure 6.5. A woman inhales and straightens her torso.

Toe, Leg, and Arm Cross

- Standing behind your chair, use your right hand to hold on to the top of your chair.

- Stand straight with your feet together.

- Breathe normally.

- Lift your left arm straight up at your left side, shoulder level (see Figure 6.6).

- Place your left foot out, shoulder width (see Figure 6.7).

- Swing your left arm to the right, past your torso (see Figure 6.8).

- Repeat three times.

- Swing your left foot past your right leg, toes touching the floor (see Figure 6.9).

- Repeat three times.

- Swing both your left arm and left foot together (see Figure 6.10).

- Repeat three times.

- Turn and face the opposite direction.

- Standing behind your chair, use your left hand to hold on to the top of your chair.

- Stand straight with your feet together.

- Breathe normally.

- Lift your right arm straight up at your right side, shoulder level.

- Place your right foot out, shoulder width.

- Swing your right arm to the left, past your torso.

- Repeat three times.

- Swing your right foot past your left leg, toes touching the floor.

- Repeat three times.

- Swing your right arm and right foot together.

- Repeat three times.

- Incorporate the song "Simple Gifts" (Fox, 1987).

- While swinging your left arm and foot, sing in a medium tempo:

> "'Tis a gift to be simple, 'tis a gift to be free,
> 'Tis a gift to come down where we ought to be."

- Turn and change directions.

- While swinging your right arm and foot, continue singing the song:

> "And when we find ourselves in the place just right,
> 'Twill be in the valley of love and delight."

- Repeat the movements with the song three times.

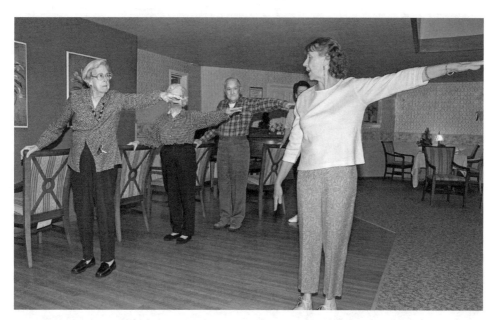

Figure 6.6. The class members lift their left arms straight at shoulder level during the Toe, Leg, and Arm Cross exercise.

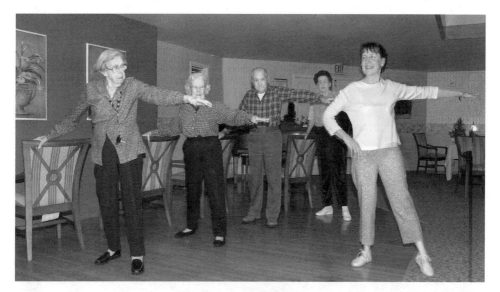

Figure 6.7. The participants place their left feet out, shoulder width.

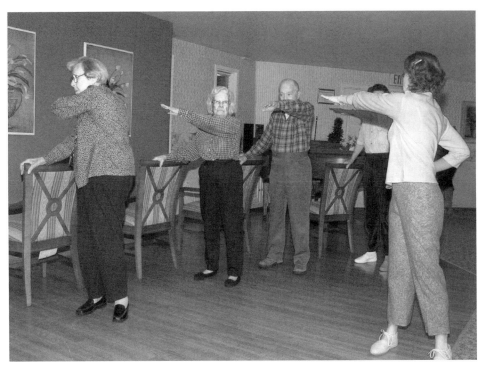

Figure 6.8. The participants swing their left arms to the right, past their torsos.

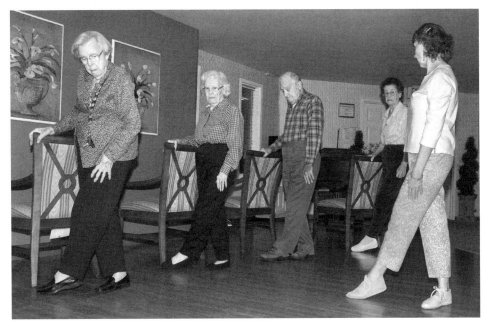

Figure 6.9. The class members swing their left feet past their right legs with their toes touching the floor.

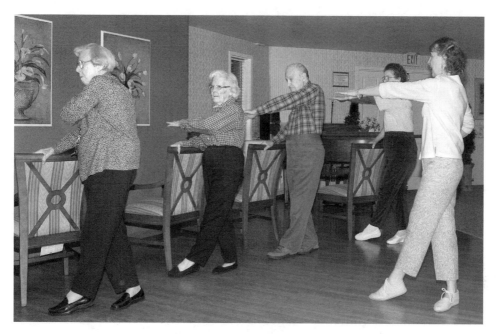

Figure 6.10. The participants swing their left arms and left feet together.

Bilateral Exercises 2a: Seated

Body Stretch

- Sit straight, with your back slightly away from your chair (see Figure 6.11).

- Place both feet apart, a little wider than the width of your hips.

- Interlace your fingers (see Figure 6.12).

- Inhale as you straighten your arms and raise them over your head (see Figure 6.13).

- Exhale and lower your arms to shoulder height with your fingers interlaced (see Figure 6.14).

- Inhale and move your arms to the right with your fingers interlaced (see Figure 6.15).

- Exhale and come back to center.

- Inhale and move your arms to the left with your fingers interlaced.

- Exhale and come back to center.

- Keep fingers interlaced, inhale, and raise your arms straight over your head (see Figure 6.16).

- Exhale, lowering your head, torso, and arms to the floor (see Figure 6.17).

- Inhale and slowly raise your head, torso, and arms (see Figure 6.18).

- Release your fingers, and place your hands on your knees (see Figure 6.19)

- Repeat three times.

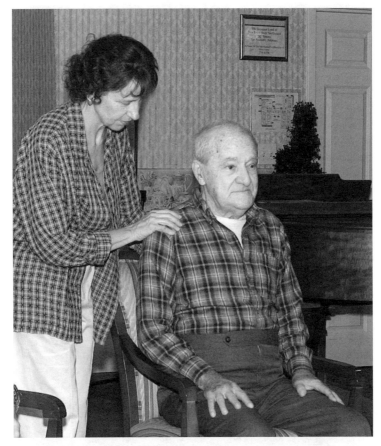

Figure 6.11. This man sits straight with his back slightly away from the chair to begin the Body Stretch sequence.

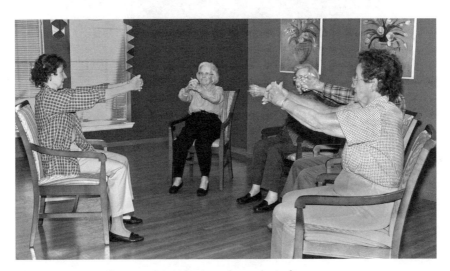

Figure 6.12. The participants interlace their fingers.

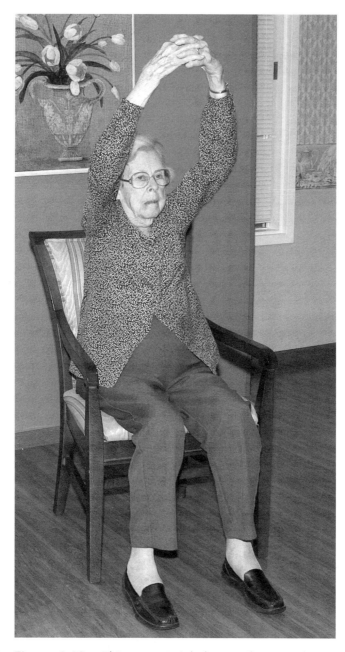

Figure 6.13. This woman inhales as she straightens her arms and raises them over her head.

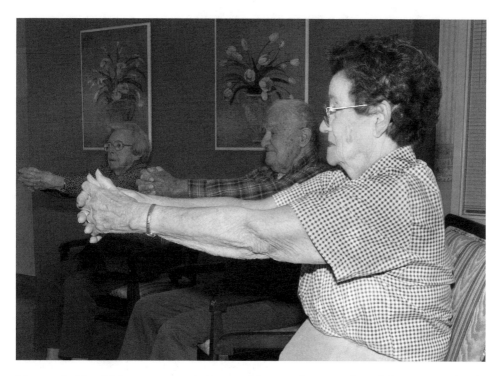

Figure 6.14. This woman exhales and lowers her interlaced fingers to shoulder height.

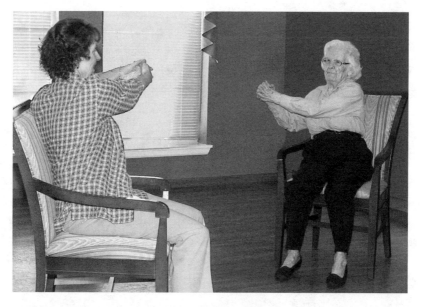

Figure 6.15. The instructor and participant inhale and rotate their arms, with fingers interlaced, to the right.

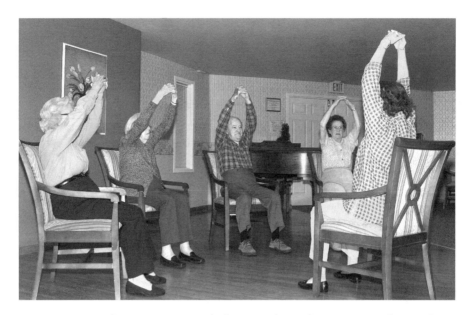

Figure 6.16. The participants inhale, straighten their arms, and raise them over their heads.

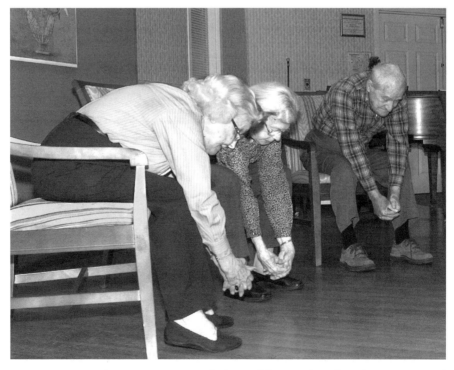

Figure 6.17. The participants exhale and lower their heads, torsos, and arms to the floor.

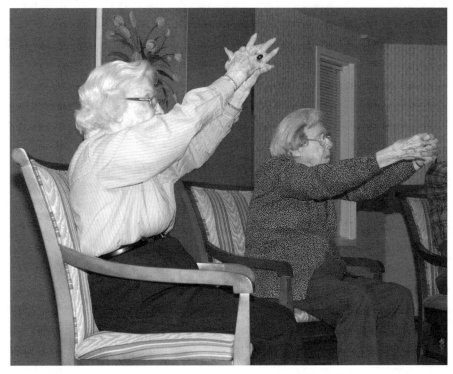

Figure 6.18. The participants inhale and slowly raise their heads, torsos, and arms.

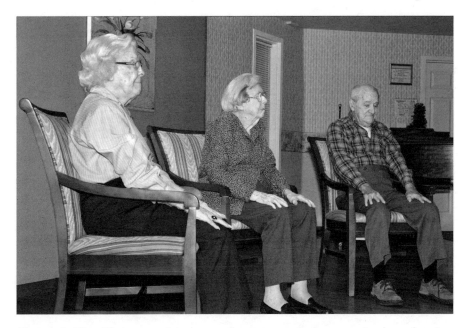

Figure 6.19. These participants prepare to end the exercise by releasing their fingers and placing their hands on their knees.

Ankle–Knee Slaps

- Sit straight, with your feet slightly apart.
- Cross your right ankle over your left knee (see Figure 6.20).
- With your left hand, slap your ankle, then your knee (see Figures 6.21 and 6.22).
- Repeat three times.
- Cross your left ankle over your right knee.
- With your right hand, slap your ankle, then your knee.
- Repeat three times.
- Incorporate the song "Sweet Betsy from Pike" (Fox, 1987).
- Cross your right ankle over your left knee, and slap your ankle and knee in tempo with the first two lines:

  "Oh, don't you remember Sweet Betsy from Pike?
  Who crossed the big mountains with her lover Ike."

- Cross your left ankle over your right knee, and slap your ankle and knee in tempo with the last two lines:

  "With two yoke of oxen, a big yaller dog,
  A tall Shanghai rooster, and one spotted hog."

- Repeat three times.

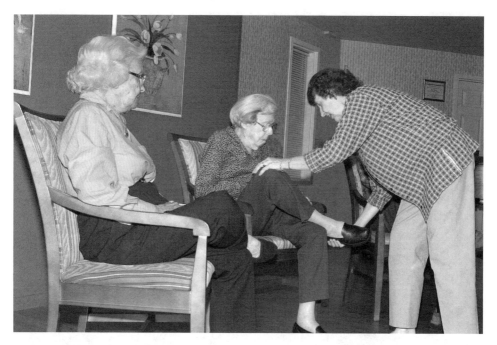

Figure 6.20. The instructor helps a woman cross her right ankle over her left knee to prepare for the Ankle–Knee Slaps.

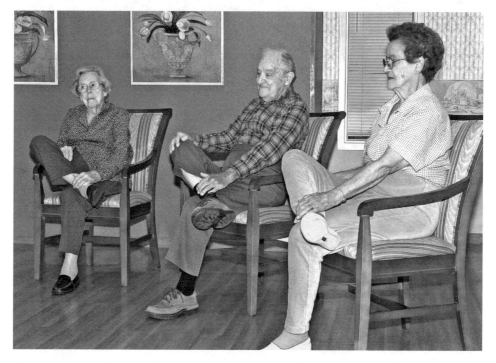

Figure 6.21. The group members slap their ankles with their left hands.

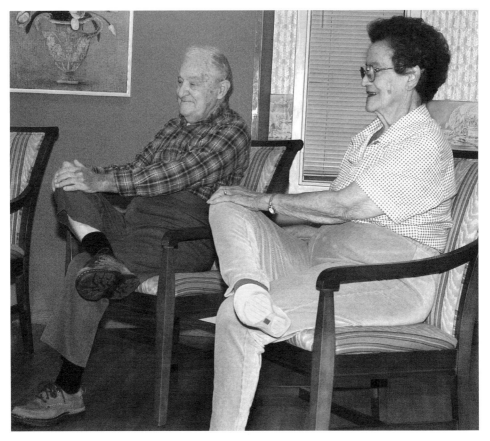

Figure 6.22. After the participants slap their ankles, they slap their knees.

Bilateral Exercises 2b: Standing

Cross-Over

- Stand facing the back of your chair.

- Hold on to the top of the chair with your right hand in front of your left leg.

- Straighten your right arm.

- Breathe normally.

- Lift your left arm in a circular motion, passing it over your head (see Figure 6.23).

- Place your left hand over your right hand on top of the chair (see Figure 6.24).

- Straighten your left arm.

- Lift your right arm in a circular motion, passing it over your head.

- Place your right hand on the top of the chair in front of your left leg.

- Repeat sequence five times.

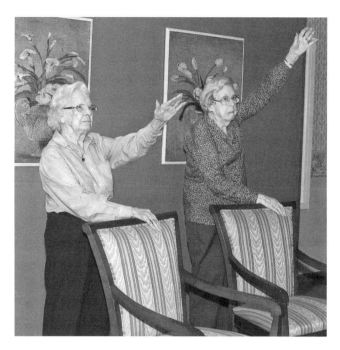

Figure 6.23. These women lift their left arms in a circular motion, passing them over their heads.

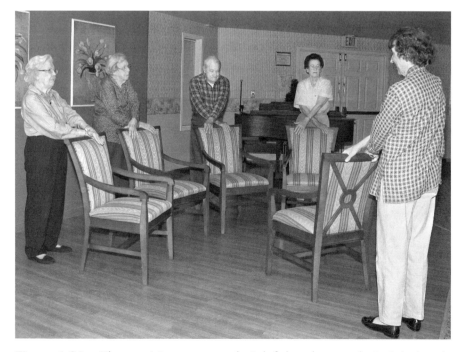

Figure 6.24. The participants cross their left hands over their right hands on the top of the chair.

Scissor Leg Lifts

- With your right hand, hold on to the top of the chair for support.

- Stand straight with your feet together and place your left hand on your hip (see Figure 6.25).

- Inhale and lift your left leg to the side (see Figure 6.26).

- Exhale and lower your left leg.

- Cross your left leg over your right leg, toes touching the floor (see Figure 6.27).

- Inhale and lift your left leg to the side.

- Exhale and lower your left leg.

- Cross your left leg behind your right leg, toes touching the floor (see Figure 6.28).

- Repeat three times.

- Turn to face the opposite direction.

- With your left hand, hold on to the top of the chair.

- Stand straight with your feet together.

- Place your right hand on your hip.

- Inhale and lift your right leg to the side.

- Exhale and lower your right leg.

- Cross your right leg over your left leg, toes touching the floor.

- Inhale and lift your right leg to the side.

- Exhale and lower your right leg.

- Cross your right leg behind your left leg, toes touching the floor.

- Repeat three times.

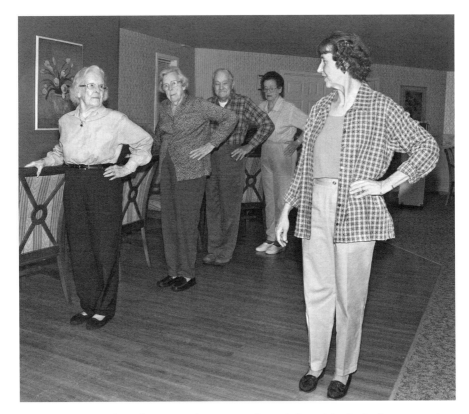

Figure 6.25. The class members stand straight with their feet together and left hands on their hips to prepare for the Scissor Leg Lifts.

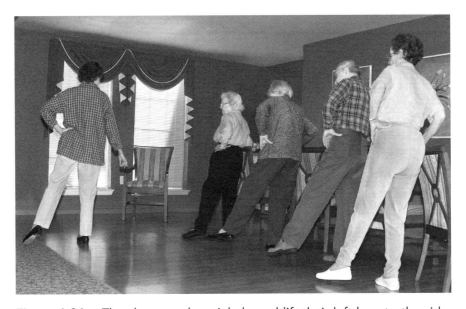

Figure 6.26. The class members inhale and lift their left legs to the side.

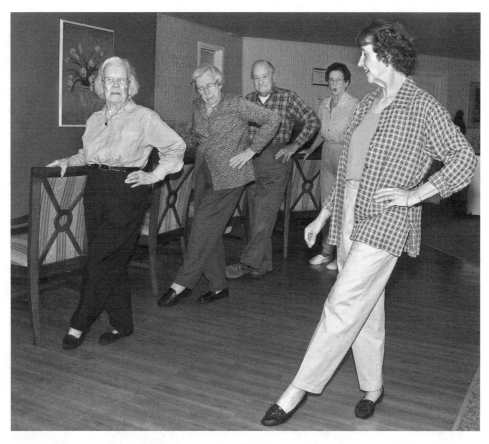

Figure 6.27. Group members cross their left legs over their right legs, toes touching the floor.

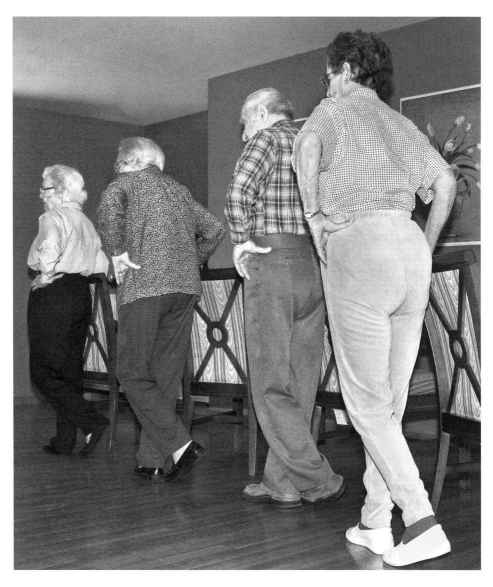

Figure 6.28.   Participants exhale and lower their left legs, crossing their left legs behind their right legs, toes touching the floor.

Movement with Meaning provides a context for people in early-stage Alzheimer's disease to experience the integration of both the mind and the body. These individuals not only need validation of their feelings and subjective experience but also require a way to come back *home*. To be able to navigate their world is crucial to foster independence and to rediscover the core of their essential being with an internal sense of feeling at *home* in their bodies. As one family caregiver stated, "I took Frank out to lunch after the class, and our friends commented on how *present* he was during our conversation." Enhancing conscious awareness, both internal and external, is one of the main objectives of Movement with Meaning.

7

Nice and Easy Yoga

"May I be at peace,
May my heart be open,
May I awaken to the light of my own true nature,
May I be healed,
May I be a source of healing for all beings."

—Loving Kindness Meditation

Yoga comes from the Sanskrit word meaning "to yoke" or "to join." The practice of yoga postures began thousands of years ago. Bilateral in nature, the postures stimulate both the right and left hemispheres in the brain. A sense of equilibrium is enhanced when the midline of the body is in alignment with the earth.

Yoga postures increase our spatial awareness, gross motor perception, and concentration. More important, orientation to one's body in time and space is improved when yoga postures are incorporated into an exercise program.

Yoga is introduced after the memorization and visualization segment of the Movement with Meaning™ program. Therefore, what was learned by memorizing a poem or song is reinforced in the physical realm of the body, bringing the mind and body together in harmony (Khalsa &

Stauth, 1997). Furthermore, the yoga postures lessen anxiety and create a sense of validation regarding the participant's subjective experience.

Yoga develops flexibility through gentle stretching poses that create a feeling of agility, which, in turn, increases the knowledge of how the body moves and reacts. Improving agility conserves energy and promotes better coordination and balance (Small, 2002).

Individuals in early-stage Alzheimer's disease feel more comfortable when the sequence of the postures is repeated in the same way for each class. By anticipating the next pose, they can focus on the present and experience the mind–body connection (Coulter, 2001).

Most of the postures are gentle seated exercises, beginning with a series of warm-ups that include shoulder rotations, head rolls, arm circles, and elbow touches. They continue with a variety of seated postures such as simple twists, arm stretches, and leg lifts. For standing poses, participants use the back of a chair for balance and continue with leg lifts and the supported standing reach pose.

The participants strive for fluidity when moving from one pose to the next. The poses become second nature to the participants as each sequence is sustained by repetition (Mehta, Mehta, & Mehta, 1990). In a subtle way, the postures have a rhythmic sense of their own, ebbing and flowing. This allows each participant to become focused in the present as the postures work within a system of synchronized movements.

As mentioned in Chapter 6, the bilateral exercises and the yoga postures can be interchanged. I suggest, for the sake of continuity, choosing either the bilateral exercises or the yoga postures for the same class program until you and the participants agree to begin a new class, introducing a different breathing technique with a new poem or song.

SEGMENT 3B

YOGA POSTURES

Be aware of the seating arrangements before beginning the yoga postures. The chairs should be a comfortable distance from one another to allow space for arm and leg movements. Introduce this segment by asking the participants if they are familiar with yoga postures. If anyone has had some experience with yoga, invite him or her to briefly talk about it. In a gentle way, try to focus discussion on the benefits of yoga—how it works to lessen anxiety and confusion while increasing concentration and balance.

Begin by demonstrating each posture two or three times while you verbally explain how each posture is done. Take your time and speak slowly and clearly, making sure that each participant can see and hear you.

Yoga Warm-Ups 1 (Seated Postures)

Shoulder Rotations

- Sit with your back straight and arms at your sides (see Figure 7.1).

- Lift your shoulders and roll them up, back, down, and forward (see Figure 7.2).

- Repeat three times.

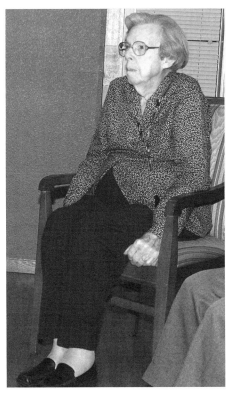

Figure 7.1. A participant sits with her back straight, arms at her sides.

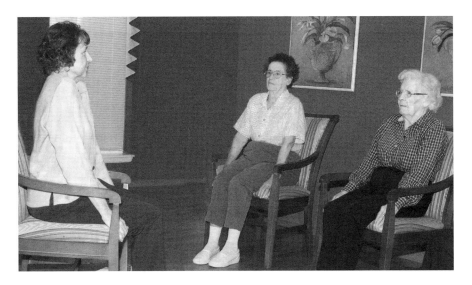

Figure 7.2. Participants lift their shoulders and roll them up, back, down, and forward.

Elbow Touch

- Sit with your back straight and your feet pointed straight ahead.

- Lift your elbows to shoulder height, placing your fingertips on your shoulders with your arms spread wide (see Figure 7.3).

- Exhale and touch your elbows together (see Figure 7.4).

- Inhale and move your elbows back.

- Repeat five times.

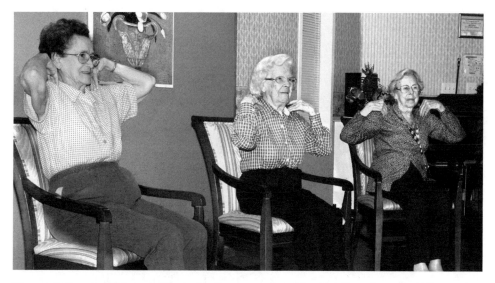

Figure 7.3. Participants lift their elbows to shoulder height, place their fingertips on their shoulders, and spread their arms wide.

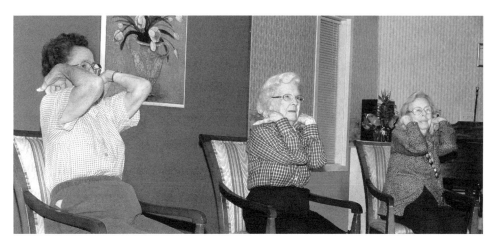

Figure 7.4. Participants exhale and touch their elbows together.

Yoga Seated Leg and Arm Postures 1

Leg Lifts (seated)

- With your back straight, place your hands on your lap or on the sides of your chair.

- Exhale completely.

- Inhale and lift your right leg straight ahead, foot flexed (see Figure 7.5).

- Exhale and lower your leg.

- Inhale and lift your left leg straight ahead, foot flexed.

- Exhale and lower your leg.

- Repeat three times.

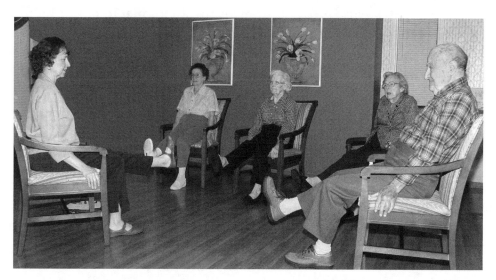

Figure 7.5. Participants inhale and lift their right legs straight ahead, feet flexed.

Sun Salutation

- Sit with your back straight and your hips back against the chair.

- Place your legs hip-distance apart, and point your feet straight ahead (see Figure 7.6).

- Exhale completely.

- Inhale and circle your arms out and up until they are over your head (see Figure 7.7).

- Look up, and place your hands together.

- Exhale and bring your chin to your chest.

- Bend over and bring your arms between your legs, placing your hands on the floor (see Figure 7.8).

- Inhale and circle your arms up again, placing your hands together (see Figure 7.9).

- Exhale and circle your arms down to your lap (see Figure 7.10).

- Repeat five times.

- Incorporate the following poem:

> "The pedigree of honey
> Does not concern the bee;
> A clover, any time, to him
> Is aristocracy."
> —Emily Dickinson (Todd & Higginson, 1982)

- Repeat the poem two times.

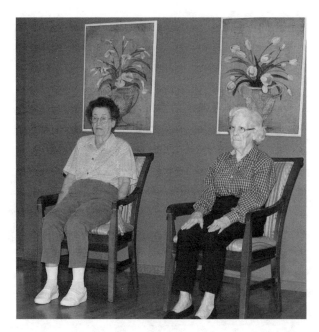

Figure 7.6. Participants place their legs hip-distance apart and point their feet straight ahead.

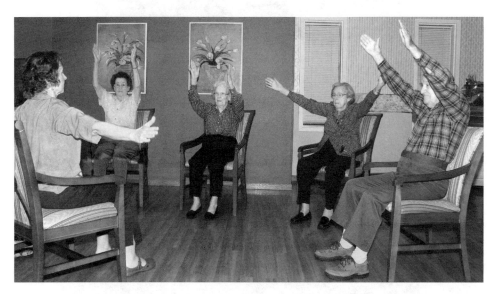

Figure 7.7. Participants inhale and circle their arms out and up until over heads.

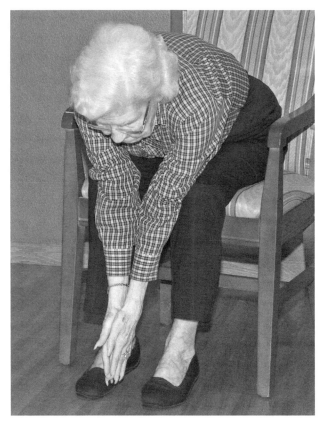

Figure 7.8. A woman bends over and brings her arms between her legs.

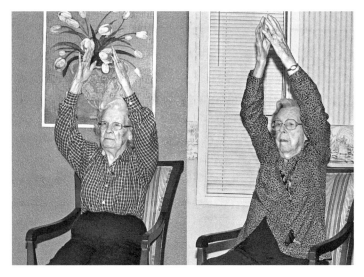

Figure 7.9. Participants inhale and circle their arms up again, placing their hands together.

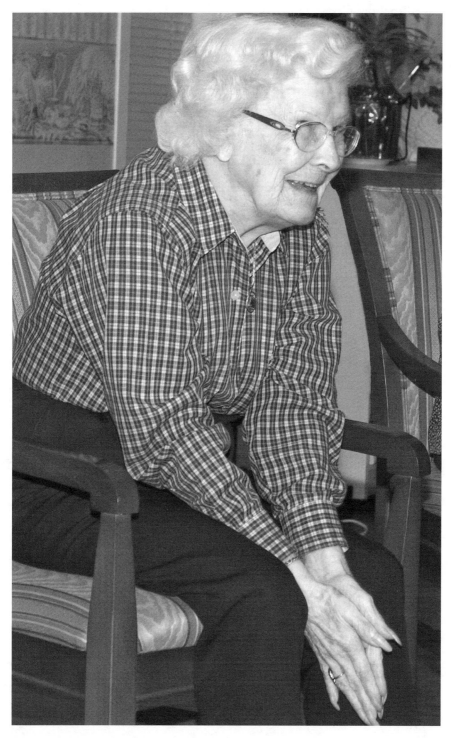

Figure 7.10. A woman exhales and circles her arms down to her lap.

Leg Lifts (standing)

- With your right hand, hold on to the top of the chair.
- Stand straight, feet slightly apart (see Figure 7.11).
- Exhale completely.
- Inhale and lift your right leg (see Figure 7.12).
- Exhale and lower your right leg.
- Repeat three times.
- Turn and face the opposite direction.
- With your left hand, hold on to the top of the chair.
- Stand straight, feet slightly apart.
- Exhale completely.
- Inhale and lift your left leg.
- Exhale and lower your left leg.
- Repeat three times.

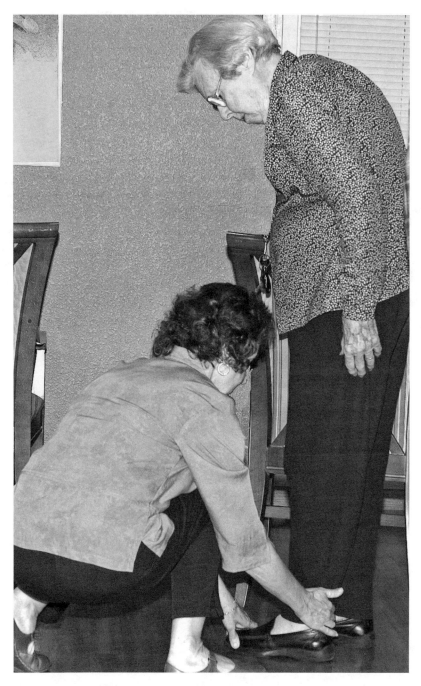

Figure 7.11. The instructor helps a woman to stand straight with her feet slightly apart.

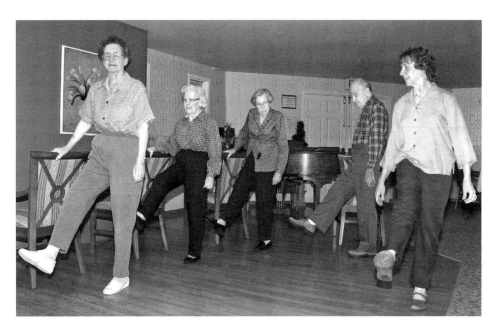

Figure 7.12. Participants inhale and lift their right legs.

Reach Pose

- With your right hand, hold on to the top of the chair.
- Exhale completely.
- Inhale and rise up on your toes (see Figure 7.13).
- Raise your left arm straight up above your head (see Figure 7.14).
- Exhale and lower your feet and arms.
- Repeat three times.
- Turn to face the opposite direction.
- With your left hand, hold on to the top of the chair.
- Exhale completely.
- Inhale and rise up on your toes.
- Raise your right arm straight up above your head.
- Exhale and lower your feet and arms.
- Repeat three times.

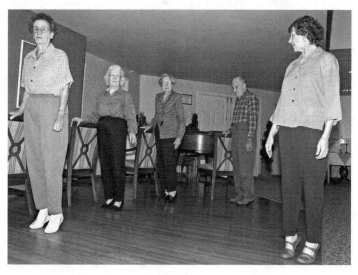

Figure 7.13.   Participants inhale and rise up on their toes.

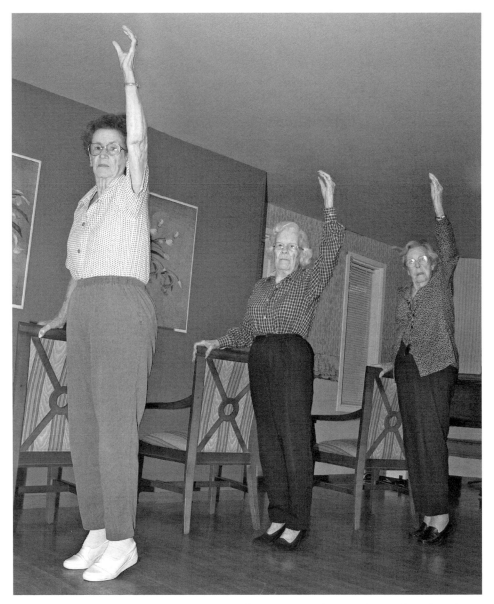

Figure 7.14.   Participants raise their left arms straight up above their heads.

Yoga Warm-Ups 2 (Seated Postures)

Head Rolls

- Place your hands in your lap (see Figure 7.15).
- Relax your shoulders.
- Breathe naturally.
- Relax your head, looking straight ahead.
- Gently bend your head forward.
- Bring your head back, looking straight ahead.
- Slowly rotate your head to the left side so that your ear is over your shoulder (see Figure 7.16).
- Bring your head back to center.
- Slowly rotate your head to the right side so that your ear is over your shoulder.
- Bring your head back to center.
- Repeat five times.

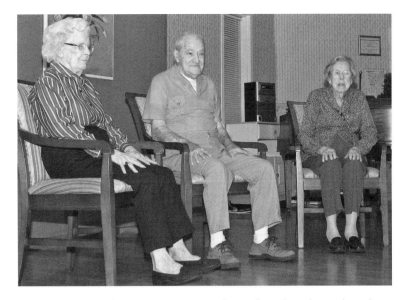

Figure 7.15. Three participants place their hands in their laps at the beginning of the Head Rolls exercise.

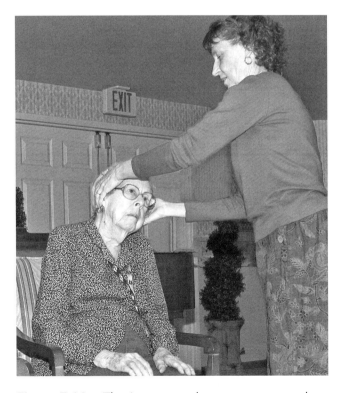

Figure 7.16. The instructor shows one woman how to slowly rotate her head to the left side so that her ear is over her shoulder.

Stretch with Tie

- Hold a tie pulled tight at each end.

- Straighten your arms, and place the tie on your lap (see Figure 7.17).

- Maintain tension between your hands.

- Begin by raising your arms slowly, inhaling, until your arms are overhead (see Figures 7.18 and 7.19).

- Exhale and bring your arms slowly down to your lap (see Figure 7.20).

- Repeat five times.

- Incorporate the following poem:

> "To see a World in a Grain of Sand
> And a Heaven in a Wild Flower,
> Hold Infinity in the palm of your hand
> And Eternity in an hour."
> —William Blake (Kazin, 1968)

- Repeat the poem two times.

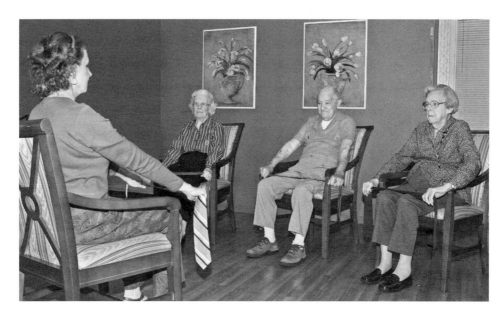

Figure 7.17.   Participants straighten their arms and place their ties on their laps.

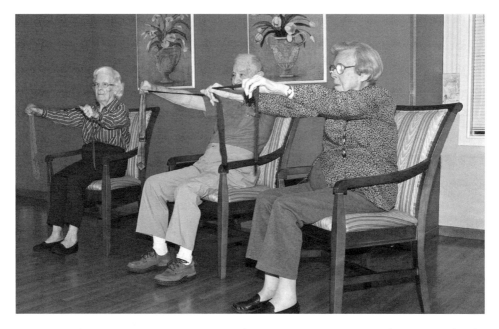

Figure 7.18.   Maintaining tension on the tie participants raise their arms slowly as they inhale.

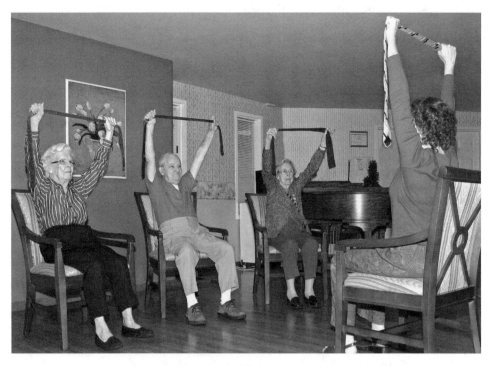

Figure 7.19. Participants raise their arms slowly until over their heads.

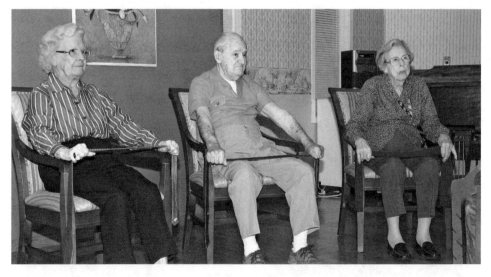

Figure 7.20. Participants exhale and slowly bring their arms down to their laps.

Side Stretch

- Sit with your feet slightly apart.

- Inhale and raise your arms out to your sides at shoulder height (see Figure 7.21).

- Exhale and bend toward the left, keeping your arms and back straight (see Figure 7.22).

- Inhale and return arms to center.

- Exhale and bend toward the right, keeping your arms and back straight.

- Inhale and return arms to center (see Figure 7.23).

- Repeat three times.

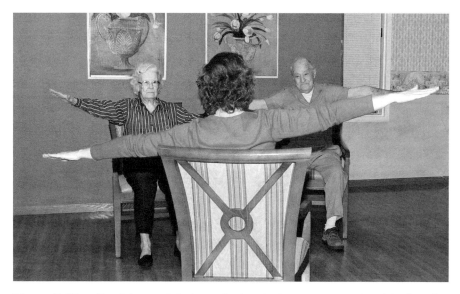

Figure 7.21.   Participants inhale and raise their arms out at shoulder height.

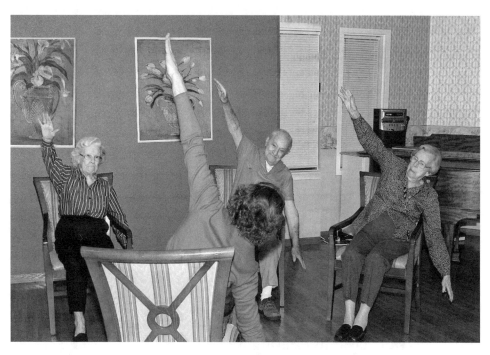

Figure 7.22. Participants exhale and bend toward the left, keeping their arms and backs straight.

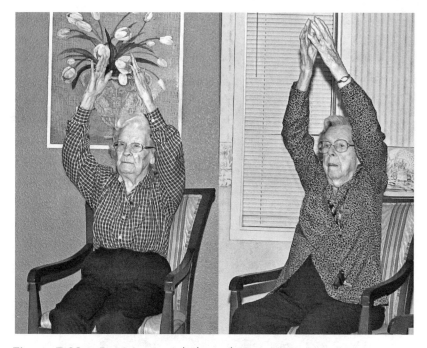

Figure 7.23. Participants inhale and return arms to center.

Knee Squeeze

- Sit with your feet slightly apart (see Figure 7.24).

- Exhale completely.

- Inhale and lift your right leg with both hands under your knee (see Figure 7.25).

- Gently pull your right knee toward your chest, tucking your head in.

- Exhale and release.

- Inhale and lift your left leg with both hands under your knee.

- Gently pull your left knee toward your chest, tucking your head in (see Figure 7.26).

- Exhale and release.

- Repeat three times.

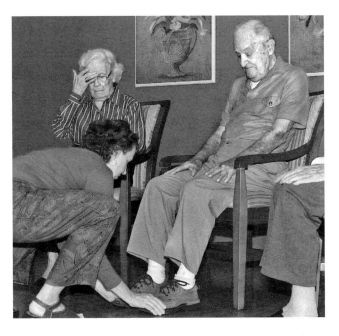

Figure 7.24. The instructor helps a participant place his feet slightly apart.

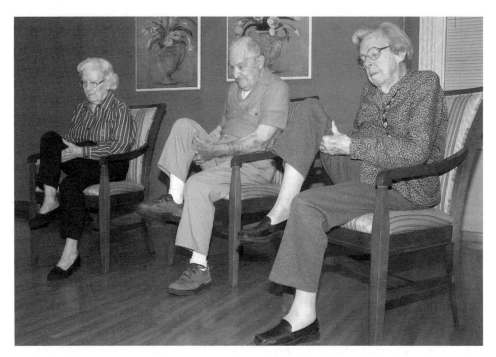

Figure 7.25.   Participants inhale and lift their right legs with both hands under their right knees.

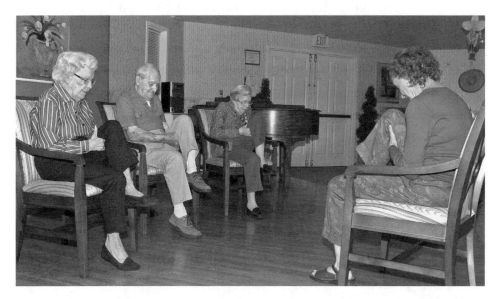

Figure 7.26.   Participants gently pull their left knees toward their chests, tucking their heads in.

Side Leg Lifts

- With your right hand, hold on to the top of your chair (see Figure 7.27).

- Stand straight with your feet together.

- Place your left hand on your hip (see Figure 7.28).

- Exhale completely.

- Inhale and lift your left leg up to the side (see Figure 7.29).

- Exhale and lower your leg.

- Repeat three times.

- Turn and face the opposite direction.

- With your left hand, hold on to the top of your chair.

- Place your right hand on your hip.

- Exhale completely.

- Inhale and lift your right leg up to the side.

- Exhale and lower your leg.

- Repeat three times.

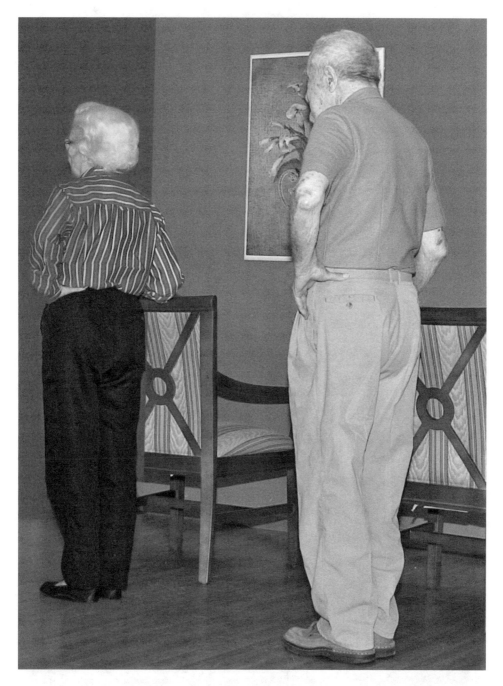

Figure 7.27. Participants hold on to the top of their chairs with their right hands.

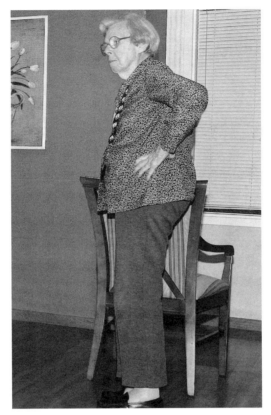

Figure 7.28. A woman demonstrates placing her left hand on her hip.

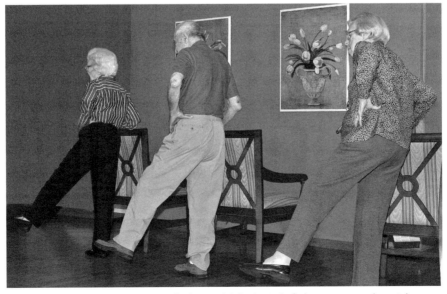

Figure 7.29. Participants inhale and lift their left legs up to the side.

Chair Twist

- With your right hand, hold on to the top of your chair.
- Stand straight with your feet together.
- Exhale completely.
- Inhale and lift your left arm over your head (see Figure 7.30).
- Exhale and slowly twist your torso to the right (see Figure 7.31).
- Inhale and twist your torso back to center (see Figure 7.32).
- Lower your left arm.
- Repeat three times.
- Turn and face the opposite direction.
- With your left hand, hold on to top of your chair.
- Stand straight with your feet together.
- Exhale completely.
- Inhale and lift your right arm over your head.
- Exhale and slowly twist your torso to the left.
- Inhale and twist your torso back to center.
- Lower your right arm.
- Repeat three times.

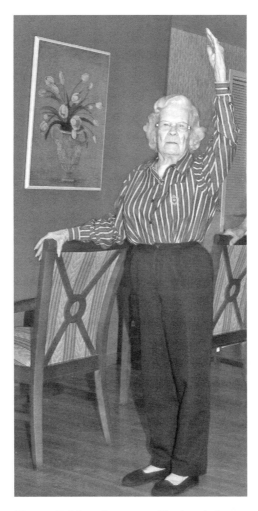

Figure 7.30.   A woman lifts her left arm over her head.

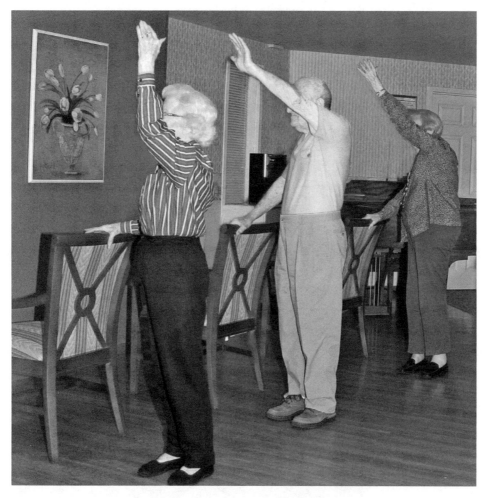

Figure 7.31. Participants exhale and slowly twist their torsos to the right.

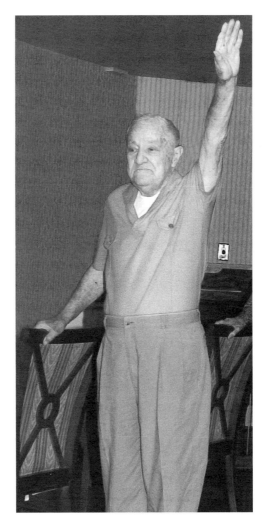

Figure 7.32. A man twists his torso back to center.

It is important to remember that there are many ways to practice yoga. Whatever method you decide to use, let it be personal. In other words, if you are enthusiastic about yoga, the participants will join you in affirming your shared experiences.

Yoga has deepened my ability to witness the process of these individuals reconnecting to their physical environment. Over time, these postures provide a true homecoming for the comfort and vitality of their bodies.

8

A Sense of Timing

"I celebrate myself, and sing myself."

—Walt Whitman (1855)

We are surrounded by music and rhythm in the natural world. Songbirds give us their distinct melodies, the seasons change, and the sun rises and sets each day. As living organisms, we human beings share our own naturally ordered rhythmic patterns. The tempo of our respiration, heartbeat, and pulse rate is individual, yet universal, in nature. On a personal level, the way in which we walk, speak, and move our bodies is especially unique.

When the effects of early-stage Alzheimer's disease begin to manifest themselves, problems with language and organization of body movements become noticeable. The individual may not be able to find the right word and say, "You know, that thing outside," when referring to a specific object such as a lawn mower or a rake. Speech is clear, but the description of things is less precise and informative (Tappen, 1997). The person may not remember the name or storyline of last night's musical number but may start to sing "I Could Have Danced All Night," and he or she will join in every verse (Arst, 1997). Although disorientation to time and space becomes evident in the early stage of

Alzheimer's disease, an individual may still show a natural rhythmic gait and motor flexibility. Just play a Glenn Miller tune, and watch how familiar music can transcend anxiety and self-consciousness.

In Movement with Meaning™, music and rhythmic exercises are used to help the participants integrate and embody a poem or song (Mathews, Clair, & Kosloski, 2001). The rhythm patterns are synchronized with the cadence and melody of the poem or song. Rhythmic instruments—such as chimes, drums, bells, and claves—are nonverbal ways of communicating. The repetition of a beat or dance evokes an inner musical sense, an inner timing. Without thinking, the participants begin to tap their feet or sway their bodies from side to side.

The movements in this segment involve our kinesthetic or "muscle" memory (Aldridge, 1994). By imitating rhythmic patterns, the body recognizes these familiar movements because they are universal in nature. Rediscovering kinesthetic memories reinforces attention and concentration, adding yet another modality to heighten awareness.

SEGMENT 4

MUSIC, RHYTHM, AND MOVEMENT

Be sure to have the necessary instruments and audiotapes or CDs close at hand before each class. Rehearse the poem or song before incorporating the instrumental or dance activity. Participants feel more relaxed and open when moving from a familiar segment to a new activity. The sequencing of the movement exercises reinforces and helps integrate the timing of the kinesthetic memory.

Poetry and Rhythm

Rhythm sticks, or claves (from Latin America), are wooden percussion instruments. These small, rounded sticks are easy to hold and simple to play. Demonstrate the basic beat and show how to tap the sticks together before handing them out to the participants (see Figure 8.1).

- Give each participant two rhythm sticks, or claves.

- Have the participants tap the sticks together without any directed beat (see Figure 8.2).

- When the participants feel comfortable with the instruments, lay them aside.

- Recite the following poem together.

> "The pedigree of honey
> Does not concern the bee;
> A clover, any time, to him
> Is aristocracy."
> —Emily Dickinson (Todd & Higginson, 1982)

- Demonstrate a slow, steady beat while incorporating the poem.

- Recite the poem while tapping the sticks together (see Figure 8.3). A natural rhythm will begin to emerge.

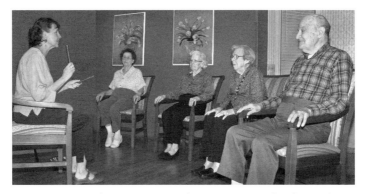

Figure 8.1. The instructor demonstrates the basic beat and shows how to tap a rhythm with the sticks.

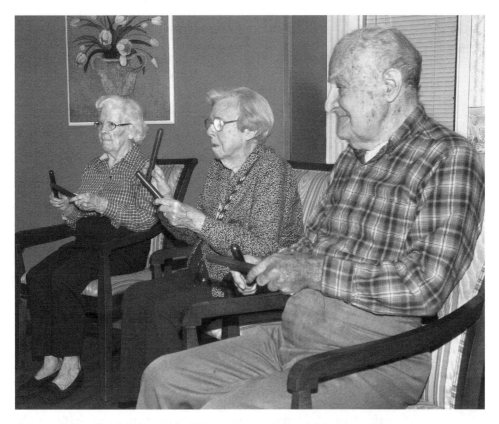

Figure 8.2. Participants tap the sticks together without a directed beat.

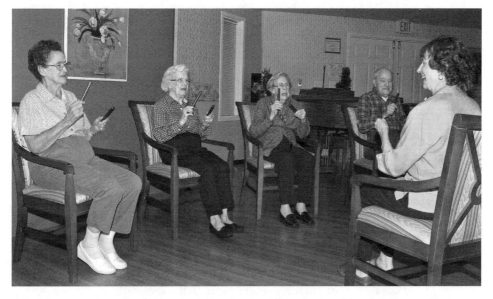

Figure 8.3. Participants recite the poem while tapping the sticks together.

Simple Song, Simple Dance

When combining a song with dance, you may want to play a soft rendition of the song in the background. The audiotape or CD can be either vocal or instrumental. The dance step is an easy two-step.

- Begin by revisiting the song "Simple Gifts" (Fox, 1987):

  "'Tis a gift to be simple, 'tis a gift to be free,
  'Tis a gift to come down where we ought to be,
  And when we find ourselves in the place just right,
  'Twill be in the valley of love and delight."

- Sing the song together a couple of times.

- Ask the participants to sing the song while you demonstrate the dance steps.

- Bring your right foot forward (see Figure 8.4).

- Bring your left foot forward, next to your right foot (see Figure 8.5).

- With feet together, bring your right foot back (see Figure 8.6).

- Bring your left foot back, next to your right foot (see Figure 8.7).

- Repeat several times, beginning with your right foot.

- Swing both arms forward and up while stepping forward (see Figure 8.8).

- Swing both arms down next to your body while stepping back (see Figure 8.9).

- Ask participants to join you by forming a circle.

- Join hands.

- Review the dance steps without the song.

- Begin to incorporate the song with the dance steps.

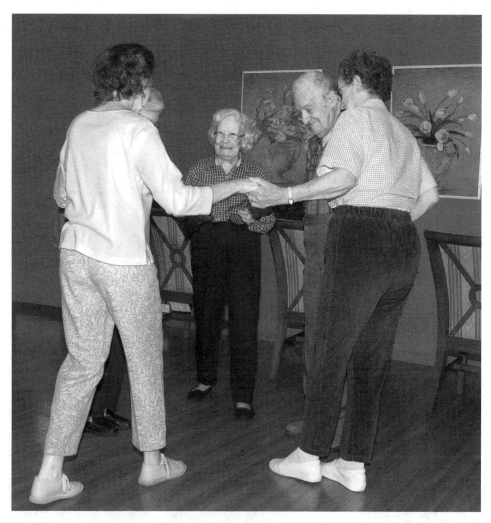

Figure 8.4. Participants bring their right feet forward in a circle dance.

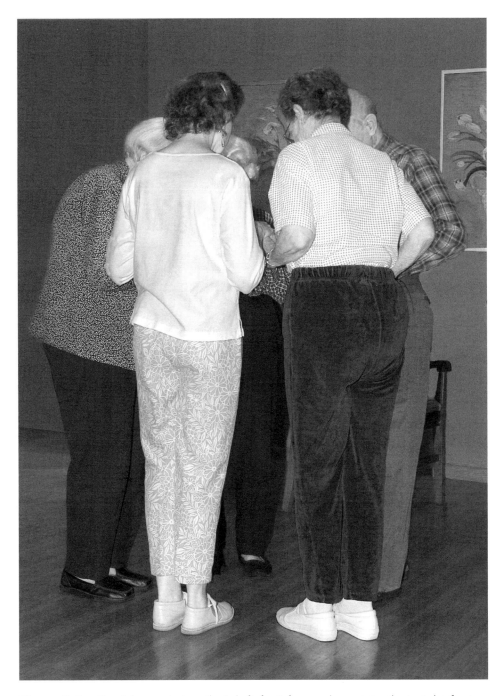

Figure 8.5. Participants bring their left feet forward, next to their right feet.

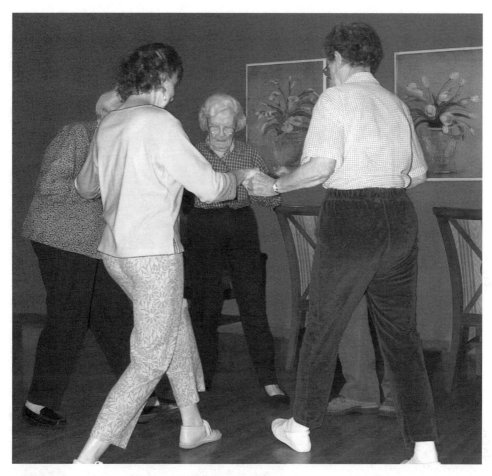

Figure 8.6. With their feet together, participants step back with their right feet.

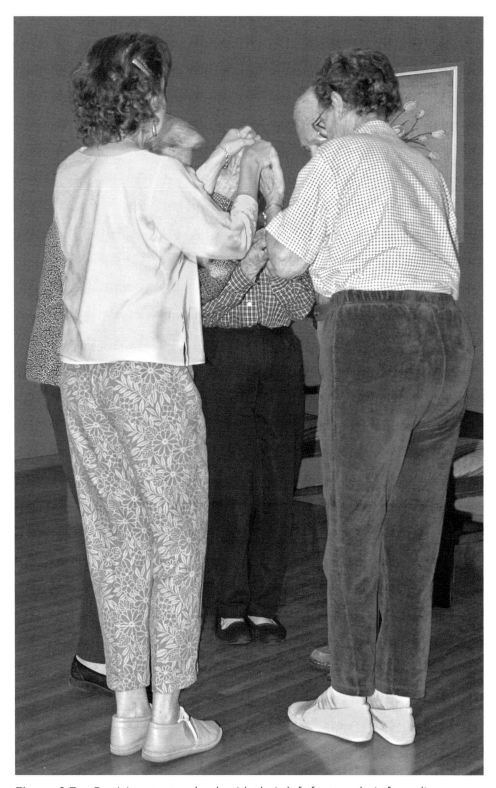

Figure 8.7. Participants step back with their left feet so their feet align.

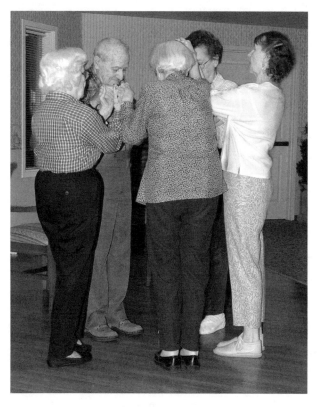

Figure 8.8.   Participants swing both arms forward and up while stepping forward.

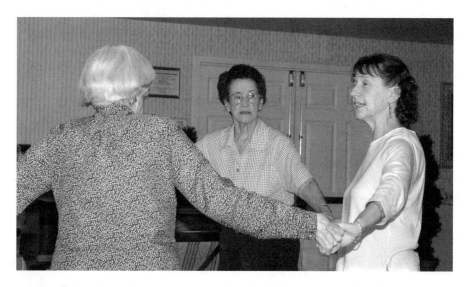

Figure 8.9.   Participants swing both arms down next to their bodies while stepping back.

Poetry and Music

Keep a variety of rhythm instruments in a wicker basket: shakers, bells, triangles, sand blocks, chimes, and claves. Demonstrate how each instrument is played before asking the participants to pick an instrument from the basket.

- Allow each participant to become acquainted with the instrument he or she chooses (see Figure 8.10).

- When the participants feel comfortable with the instruments they have selected, lay the instruments aside.

- Recite the following poem together:

> "To see a World in a Grain of Sand
> And a Heaven in a Wild Flower,
> Hold Infinity in the palm of your hand
> And Eternity in an hour."
> —William Blake (Kazin, 1968)

- Ask the participants to listen while you recite the poem with a distinct cadence, emphasizing the words *see, world, grain, sand, heaven, flower, infinity, palm, hand, eternity,* and *hour.*

- Together, recite the poem slowly with an accent on the emphasized words.

- Demonstrate how each instrument is played when the accented words are said.

- When the poem and rhythm are synchronized, play three more rounds.

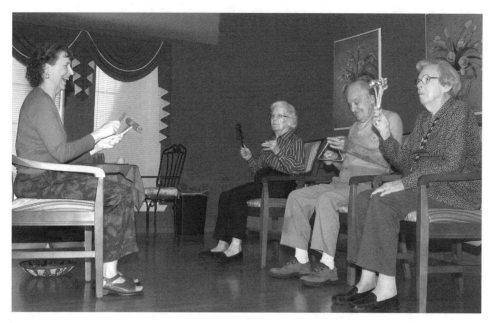

Figure 8.10. Participants become acquainted with an instrument.

Circle Dance with Betsy

This dance can be accompanied with recorded music or simply with an *a cappella* song. The tempo is a steady four- or eight-count beat, depending on the group's level of motor development.

- Begin by revisiting the song "Sweet Betsy from Pike" (Fox, 1987):

  "Oh, don't you remember Sweet Betsy from Pike?
  Who crossed the big mountains with her lover Ike.
  With two yoke of oxen, a big yaller dog,
  A tall Shanghai rooster, and one spotted hog."

- Sing the song together a couple of times.

- Ask the participants to sing the song while you demonstrate the circle dance.

- Step in to a count of four, lifting your arms (see Figure 8.11).

- Step out to a count of four, lowering your arms.

- Circle to the right to a count of four (see Figure 8.12).

- Circle to the left to a count of four (see Figure 8.13).

- Ask the participants to join you in forming a circle.

- Join hands.

- Review the steps without the song.

- Begin to incorporate the song with the circle dance.

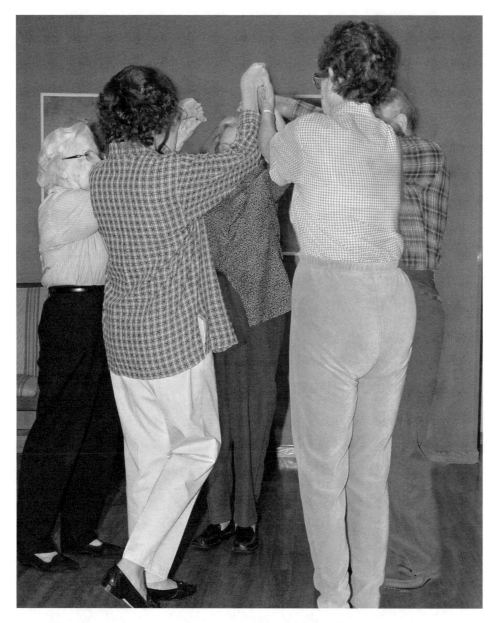

Figure 8.11. Participants step in to a count of four, lifting their arms.

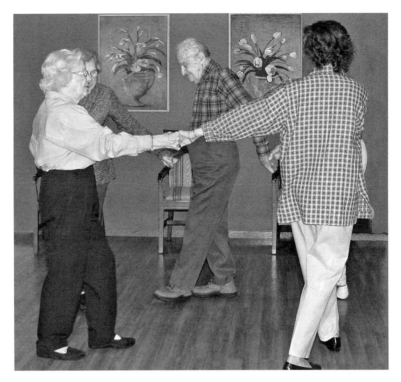

Figure 8.12.   Participants circle to the right to a count of four.

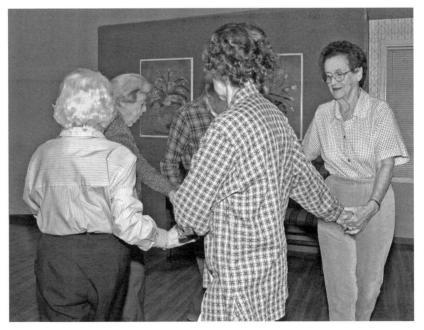

Figure 8.13.   Participants circle to the left to a count of four.

Music and dance are universal ways to celebrate the human spirit. The present becomes more vivid when individuals with Alzheimer's disease can experience their own sense of timing and creative self-expression. To be able to sing, play percussion instruments, and dance in a safe environment increases people's ability to focus and concentrate (Hill, 1999). I have witnessed the exhilaration participants feel when recovering a lost poem or song. It is as if their spirits are calling out, "I'm here, please see me!"

9

Reawakening the Senses

"Music, when soft voices die,
Vibrate in the memory;
Odours, when sweet violets sicken,
Live within the sense that quicken."

—Percy Shelley (Gardner, 1973)

Whenever I smell the scent of gardenia, my mind journeys back to a vision of my mother splashing on White Shoulders cologne before going out to dinner or a movie. I remember her so exquisitely—I sat on the bed watching her straighten the collar of her white blouse while smiling at me in the mirror. A wealth of associations are triggered from one pure scent (Erickson & Leide, 1992).

Exploring the senses allows individuals with Alzheimer's disease to gain access to their own unique internal landscapes (Feil, 2002). It is a very personal pilgrimage filled with precious memories. The last segment in Movement with Meaning™ is devoted to using the senses of smell, taste, and touch, with attention to color, shape, and texture. Therefore, the theme of each class is reinforced by yet another modality.

We make sense of the world through our senses. The body is the primary receptor and container of experience.

Our bodies perceive our environment through the senses before our minds begin to process what is happening. When we walk into a room, our bodies respond to the energy around us. Before we recognize what is going on, we find ourselves feeling calm or ill at ease.

Individuals with Alzheimer's disease begin to rely on their senses instead of their minds to interpret their environments (Burns, Byrne, & Ballard, 2002). In the middle stage of Alzheimer's disease, individuals begin to mirror their environments, taking on the moods of those around them. To generate a sense of well-being and appropriateness, they mimic the emotional energy surrounding them. For the sake of integrity, Movement with Meaning connects the participants directly to the wisdom of their bodies. They begin to become focused in the present moment by paying attention to their sensory experiences, triggered into conscious awareness by a scent, a taste, or a texture in their immediate environments (Bakker, 2003).

SEGMENT 5

FINDING SOLACE
THROUGH THE SENSES

A comfortable mood and tone in a Movement with Meaning class enables the participants to enjoy the simple pleasures of life. Incorporating sensory stimulation techniques arouses and promotes curiosity. Rekindling the senses sparks treasured memories while increasing sensory awareness (Brackey, 2000).

The Pedigree of Honey, Honey

Have a serving plate, crackers, and a jar of honey with a plastic self-pouring lid available. This activity reinforces the theme of the Emily Dickinson poem memorized at the beginning of class.

- Begin by reciting the poem together:

> "The pedigree of honey
> Does not concern the bee;
> A clover, any time, to him
> Is aristocracy."
> —Emily Dickinson (Todd & Higginson, 1982)

- Spread the crackers on a serving plate.

- Give the serving plate to a participant.

- Pour a little honey on a cracker (see Figure 9.1).

- Direct the first participant to pour honey on a cracker (see Figure 9.2).

- Ask the same participant to pass the serving plate to the next participant.

- Continue until everyone has participated in pouring honey on a cracker.

- Pass the serving plate around so each participant has a cracker with honey on top.

- Ask the participants to close their eyes while eating the cracker (see Figure 9.3).

- Recite the Dickinson poem together.

- Ask participants to open their eyes and discuss memories associated with the taste of honey (see Figure 9.4).

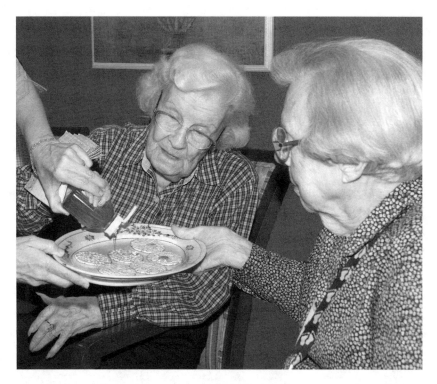

Figure 9.1. The instructor pours a little honey on a cracker.

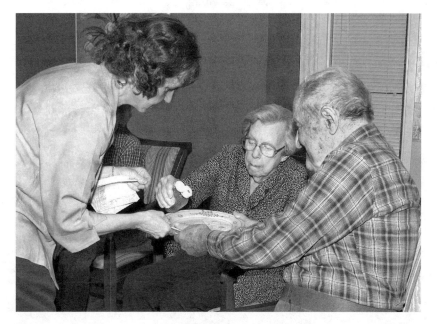

Figure 9.2. The participants are directed to pour honey on a cracker.

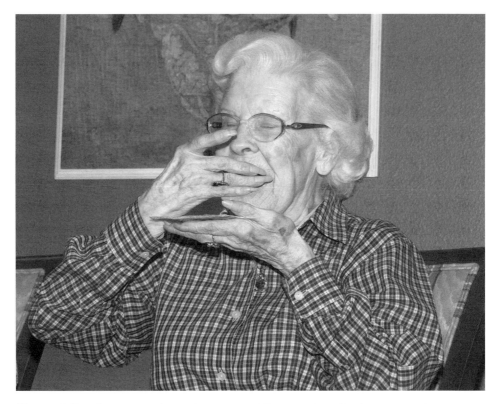

Figure 9.3. A woman closes her eyes while savoring the honey cracker.

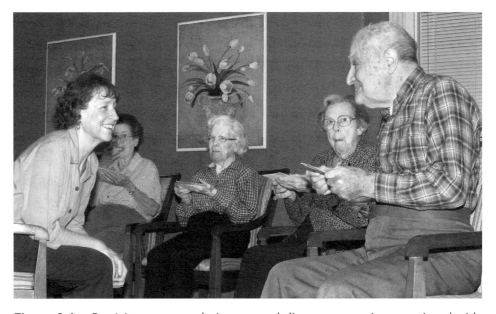

Figure 9.4. Participants open their eyes and discuss memories associated with the taste of honey.

A Simple Tea Party

Sharing a cup of tea is a way to communicate in a noninvasive, inclusive manner. For this activity, you'll need an electric teapot and a small basket of herbal teas. If at all possible, arrange a table with porcelain cups and saucers, a sugar or honey bowl, and a small pitcher for milk. Decorate the table with a light-colored tablecloth and cloth napkins.

- Revisit the song "Simple Gifts" (Fox, 1987):

  "'Tis a gift to be simple, 'tis a gift to be free,
  'Tis a gift to come down where we ought to be,
  And when we find ourselves in the place just right,
  'Twill be in the valley of love and delight."

- Ask one of the participants to turn on the electric teapot.

- Pass around the basket of herbal teas (see Figure 9.5).

- While the water is warming, ask each participant which tea he or she has chosen.

- Inquire if any of the participants have memories of tea parties from their youth.

- Pour the water in each cup with an herbal tea bag inside the cup (see Figure 9.6).

- After the tea is ready to drink, pass around the milk, sugar, and honey.

- Ask the participants to smell the aroma of the tea (see Figure 9.7).

- Ask the participants if any simple delights are recalled by the smell and taste of the tea (see Figure 9.8).

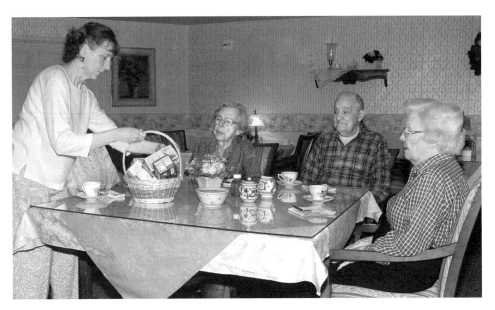

Figure 9.5.   Participants pass around a basket of herbal teas and choose one.

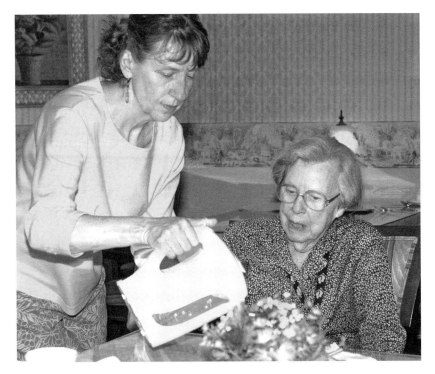

Figure 9.6.   The instructor pours water into each cup with an herbal tea bag inside.

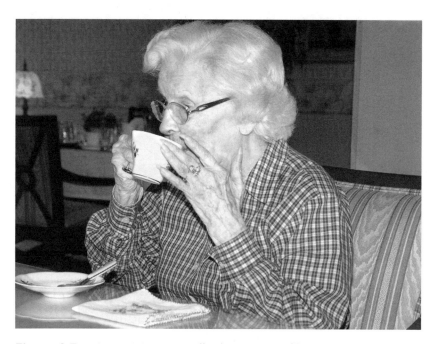

Figure 9.7. A participant smells the aroma of her tea.

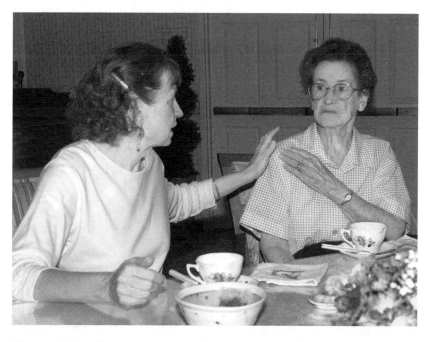

Figure 9.8. The instructor asks a woman what memories were recalled by the smell and taste of the tea.

A Grain of Sand and a Wild Flower

This activity incorporates the sense of touch with the sense of smell. Fill two plastic containers—approximately 12 inches wide by 3–4 inches deep—with sand. Place a vase filled with a variety of fragrant flowers (e.g., daisies, carnations, roses) on the table next to the containers of sand.

- Recite the following poem together:

> "To see a World in a Grain of Sand
> And a Heaven in a Wild Flower,
> Hold Infinity in the palm of your hand
> And Eternity in an hour."
> —William Blake (Kazin, 1968)

- Invite the participants to feel the sand with their fingers (see Figure 9.9).

- Ask each participant to notice the texture of the sand.

- Let each participant pick a flower from the vase (see Figure 9.10).

- Ask the participants to pay attention to the scent of their flowers (see Figure 9.11).

- Ask the participants to identify the colors and textures associated with their flowers (see Figure 9.12).

- Recite the Blake poem together.

- Have the participants close their eyes and think of the sand and their flowers.

- Ask each participant what stands out in his or her mind (e.g., color, scent, texture).

- Ask the participants to recall memories that arise from this experience (see Figure 9.13).

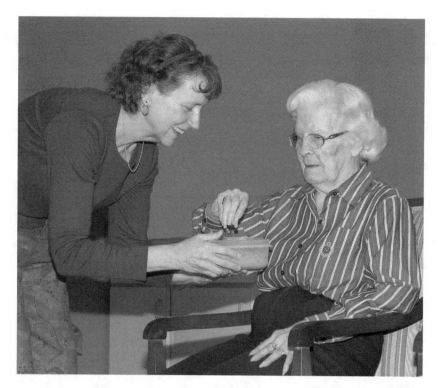

Figure 9.9. This participant is invited to feel the sand with her fingers.

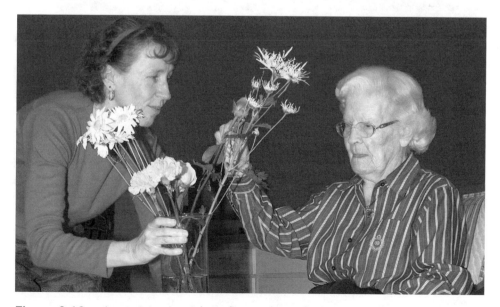

Figure 9.10. A participant picks a flower from the vase.

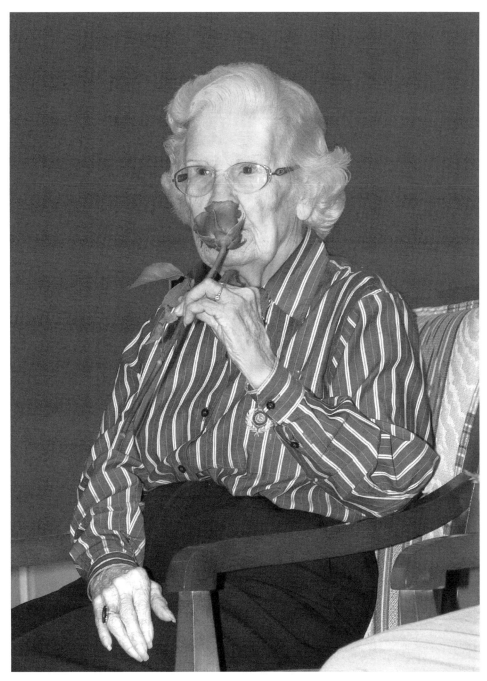

Figure 9.11.   A woman enjoys the scent of her flower.

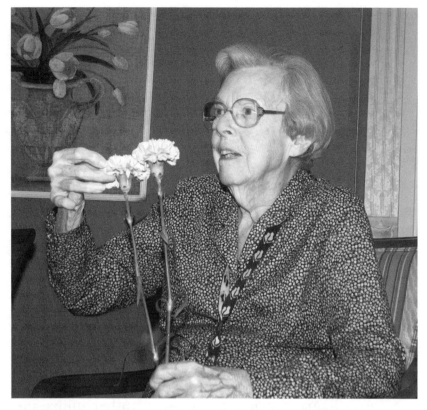

Figure 9.12. A woman identifies the colors and textures associated with her flower.

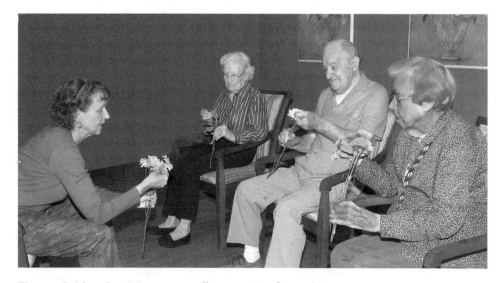

Figure 9.13. Participants recall memories from this experience.

Sweet Betsy's Animal Fair

Almost everyone had a favorite pet as a child. Before this class begins, write a note asking each participant to bring in a photograph of a beloved pet, either from childhood or any time in adult life. Bring a variety of stuffed but realistic-looking animals or large laminated animal pictures to class. To reinforce the song "Sweet Betsy from Pike," include a dog, pig, and rooster.

- Begin the class by singing "Sweet Betsy from Pike" (Fox, 1987):

  "Oh, don't you remember Sweet Betsy from Pike?
  Who crossed the big mountains with her lover Ike.
       With two yoke of oxen, a big yaller dog,
     A tall Shanghai rooster, and one spotted hog."

- Ask the participants to choose a stuffed animal or laminated animal picture (see Figure 9.14).

- Invite the participants to share any adventures they had with a childhood pet or farm animal.

- Introduce a photograph of a special animal in your life.

- Ask the participants if they would like to share a photograph of a favorite pet (see Figure 9.15).

- Give each participant the opportunity to reminisce about their beloved pet with a short story, with a particular characteristic they treasure, or just by passing around the photograph (see Figure 9.16).

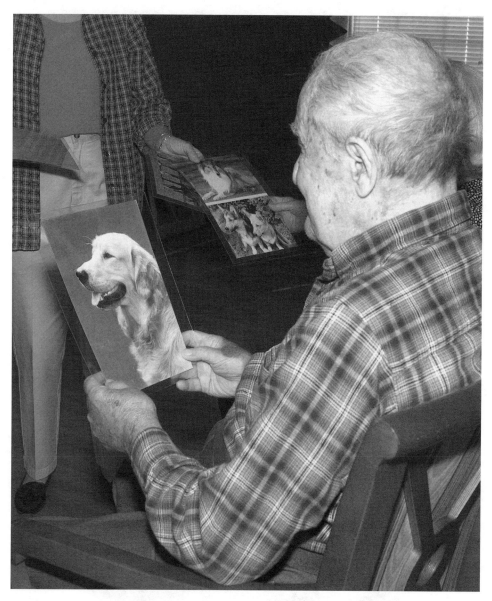

Figure 9.14. A participant chooses a laminated animal picture.

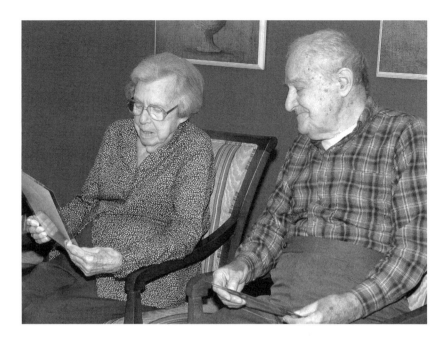

Figure 9.15.   A man and woman reminisce about the pets in their lives.

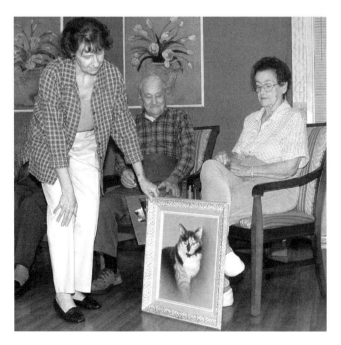

Figure 9.16.   A cat picture brings up stories from the participants' lives.

When individuals with Alzheimer's disease are not preoccupied with feeling anxious or confused, they can begin to see things they might not have noticed before. Movement with Meaning intensifies the present by embracing the rich moments in life via the senses. There is no timeline when living in the present. When life is experienced as a continuum, the past is ever present. To make sense of the world, individuals with Alzheimer's disease need an environment that engages their curiosity and, more important, expands their capacity for hope and meaning.

10

Carefully Choreographed Chaos

"When we try to pick
out anything by itself, we find it
hitched to everything else in the universe."

—John Muir (1979)

A natural blending and unfolding occur in a respectful manner in a Movement with Meaning™ class. There's no rush or hurry to get through an entire class—the participants act as a gauge to determine its pace and organic rhythm. In other words, the *process* is more important than the *product*.

Allow yourself to relax and enjoy getting acquainted with each participant on a more personal level. Intimacy is as necessary as oxygen for human beings to thrive. As Mother Teresa said, "Everyone needs to feel loved and purposeful." Movement with Meaning promises to harvest the gathered resources in an environment that gives each participant the opportunity to contribute his or her unique gifts while preserving his or her dignity and autonomy.

Bringing all of the sensory modalities into play allows the individual with Alzheimer's disease to experience an attentive relationship between the outer world and his or her inner landscape. It is therefore essential that the chore-ography in each class be practiced in a slow but conscious rhythm. It may take 3 to 4 weeks to complete an entire class, depending on how often the group meets. Ideally, a Movement with Meaning class meets over a 30-minute time frame, 3–5 days a week.

Each of the four classes presented in Movement with Meaning act as a framework on which to build. As you become more at ease with the underlying objective of the program, you can begin to interweave activities and exer-cises that are of interest to you and the participants. Each individual will demonstrate a particular fondness for poetry, music, or movement, and the group as a whole will have a preference. Don't be afraid to take healthy risks. Gather the activities together and find a theme from which to draw.

Movement with Meaning gives participants the oppor-tunity to shift focus from being captives of Alzheimer's disease to embracing their immense personal history by exploring the rich texture of their ever-present past. The mist that has engulfed the brain rises from what seemed to be a forgotten landscape, and distinct places, voices, odors, and experiences become visible and recognizable once again.

As the sequence of activities becomes familiar, a subtle understanding will begin to surface. The participants feel more confident and less anxious. As explanations fall away, there is less need for unnecessary verbiage. A sense of sacredness is expressed through the natural rhythm and choreography of the class. Let it be, and enjoy communicat-ing on a more nonverbal level.

Harmony replaces confusion and doubt. The partici-pants begin to trust their bodies to know what comes next in the sequence of activities and exercises. The body becomes their refuge. Being in the present moment feels expansive, and their sense of purpose is no longer in ques-tion.

As the participants become familiar with the multisen-sory activities and exercises, they will begin to anticipate the sequence without having to be cued or reminded. Through total immersion in and repetition of the short, concentrated physical, mental, and sensory awareness exercises, a natural rhythm or choreography will begin to emerge. Moving from one sequence to the next will take less time because there will be no need for demonstrations and practice.

When the participants feel comfortable with all of the segments in a class, encourage them to bring songs or poems that help support the particular theme. In this way, they have a sense of purpose and place—a sense of ownership.

The initial class meeting is very important to establish a warm and trusting environment. Creating sacred space is about providing a safe haven not only to deepen your connection with each participant but also to help each participant feel comfortable and safe enough to explore his or her unique skills and talents.

As the participants gather together for the first time, an inviting atmosphere with soft classical or environmental music in the background and a light scent of lavender aromatherapy greets them. During this first encounter, spend as much time as you and the participants need for introductions and a review of the Movement with Meaning philosophy. Talk about increasing memory skills, balance, and concentration, and explain how you will help each participant retrieve memories of songs, poems, and experiences from the past. Take your time, and let the organic rhythm of the first meeting set the tone for how the class will unfold.

CLASS 1

THE BEE AND THE HONEY

For the first week of this beginning class, you may work only on the mindful breathing exercise and the poem before incorporating the yoga postures. Again, let the *process* be more important than the *product*. Reinforce the idea that *we* are creating and designing *our* sacred space together.

Segment 1

Breathing Awareness

- Sit comfortably with your back straight and your feet pointing straight ahead.

- Close your eyes.

- Breathe normally, paying attention to each inhalation and exhalation.

- Begin to focus on the rhythm of your breathing.

- Silently count at the end of each out breath.

- Breathe in, breathe out—count "one."

- Breathe in, breathe out—count "two."

- Continue to count in this way up to 10.

- Repeat once.

For the first in and out breaths, count in a soft, clear voice. At the same time, remind participants to follow their own natural breathing rhythms.

Segment 2

Poem: "The Pedigree of Honey"

"The pedigree of honey
Does not concern the bee;
A clover, any time, to him
Is aristocracy."
—Emily Dickinson (Todd & Higginson, 1982)

The first time, read the poem from index cards that you have created. For the second reading, have everyone read the poem together. Read the poem several times until the participants feel comfortable with the exercise. Then gather the cards. Recite the poem line by line, asking the participants to repeat each line until they have memorized the poem.

Ask the participants to close their eyes. Then slowly read the poem. Ask the participants to be aware of any colors, shapes, feelings, or memories that may arise. After they open their eyes, ask if anyone would like to share his or her experience in a few words.

Segment 3

Yoga Postures

Discuss the benefits of yoga and how the postures work to increase concentration and balance. Remember to demonstrate the postures as a mirror image of what the participants are supposed to do with their arms and legs.

Warm-Ups 1 (Seated Postures)

Shoulder Rotations

- Sit with your back straight and arms at your sides.
- Lift your shoulders and roll them up, back, down, and forward.
- Repeat three times.

Elbow Touch

- Sit with your back straight and your feet pointed straight ahead.
- Lift your elbows to shoulder height, placing your fingertips on your shoulders with your arms spread wide.
- Exhale and touch your elbows together.
- Inhale and move your elbows back.
- Repeat five times.

Seated Leg and Arm Postures 1

Leg Lifts

- With your back straight, place your hands on your lap or on the sides of the chair.
- Exhale completely.

- Inhale and lift your right leg straight ahead, foot flexed.

- Exhale and lower your leg.

- Inhale and lift your left leg straight ahead, foot flexed.

- Exhale and lower your leg.

- Repeat three times.

Sun Salutation

- Sit with your back straight and your hips back against the chair.

- Place your legs hip-distance apart, and point your feet straight ahead.

- Exhale completely.

- Inhale and circle your arms out and up until they are over your head.

- Look up, and place your hands together.

- Exhale and bring your chin to your chest.

- Bend over and bring your arms between your legs, placing your hands on the floor.

- Inhale and circle your arms up again, placing your hands together.

- Exhale and circle your arms down to your lap.

- Repeat five times.

- Incorporate the following poem:

> "The pedigree of honey
> Does not concern the bee;
> A clover, any time, to him
> Is aristocracy."
> —Emily Dickinson (Todd & Higginson, 1982)

- Repeat the poem two times.

Standing Chair Postures 1

Leg Lifts

- With your right hand, hold on to the top of the chair.
- Stand straight, feet slightly apart.
- Exhale completely.
- Inhale and lift your right leg.
- Exhale and lower your right leg.
- Repeat three times.
- Turn and face the opposite direction.
- With your left hand, hold on to the top of the chair.
- Stand straight, feet slightly apart.
- Exhale completely.
- Inhale and lift your left leg.
- Exhale and lower your left leg.
- Repeat three times.

Reach Pose

- With your right hand, hold on to the top of the chair.
- Exhale completely.
- Inhale and rise up on your toes.
- Raise your left arm straight up above your head.
- Exhale and lower your feet and arms.
- Repeat three times.
- Turn and face the opposite direction.
- With your left hand, hold on to the top of the chair.
- Exhale completely.
- Inhale and rise up on your toes.
- Raise your right arm straight up above your head.

- Exhale and lower your feet and arms.
- Repeat three times.

Segment 4

Poetry and Rhythm

As in the development of any artistic process, you will want to enact a smooth transition in this segment, leading the participants from the known to the unknown. Take your time and sense when they are ready to incorporate this segment. Before you begin to demonstrate the basic beat using the rhythm sticks (claves) rehearse the poem one or two times.

- Give each participant two rhythm sticks, or claves.

- Have the participants tap the sticks together without any directed beat.

- When the participants feel comfortable with the instruments, lay them aside.

- Recite the following poem together:

> "The pedigree of honey
> Does not concern the bee;
> A clover, any time, to him
> Is aristocracy."
> —Emily Dickinson (Todd & Higginson, 1982)

- Demonstrate a slow, steady beat while incorporating the poem.

- Recite the poem while tapping the sticks together. A natural rhythm will begin to emerge.

Segment 5

The Pedigree of Honey, Honey

This last segment reinforces the theme in Class 1 with a taste of honey. As in the previous segments, have your materials prepared before class.

- Have a serving plate, crackers, and a jar of honey with a plastic self-pouring lid available. This activity reinforces the theme of the Emily Dickinson poem memorized at the beginning of class.

- Begin by reciting the poem together:

> "The pedigree of honey
> Does not concern the bee;
> A clover, any time, to him
> Is aristocracy."
> —Emily Dickinson (Todd & Higginson, 1982)

- Spread the crackers on a serving plate.

- Give the serving plate to a participant.

- Pour a little honey on one cracker.

- Direct the first participant to pour honey on one cracker.

- Ask the same participant to pass the serving plate to the next participant.

- Continue until everyone has participated in pouring honey on a cracker.

- Pass the serving plate around so that each participant has a cracker with honey on top.

- Ask the participants to close their eyes while eating the cracker.

- Recite the Dickinson poem together.

- Ask participants to open their eyes and discuss any memories associated with the taste of honey.

CLASS 2

DELIGHTED WITH SIMPLE GIFTS

Stay with Class 1 until the participants have explored and developed their personal stories, skills, and talents enough to achieve a feeling of fulfillment and a sense of completion. This will vary according to the temperaments of the individual participants as well as the dynamics of the group as a whole. A class may last from 1–3 months depending, too, on how often the group meets.

Introduce the theme of Class 2 at the end of your final Class 1. Explain the title of Class 2: "Delighted with Simple Gifts." Life is full of simple gifts. As you witness the unique talents and abilities of each participant, share these observations with the class. Reassure the participants that the pace of the next class will be geared to what feels comfortable to them. Stress that the foremost objective is for each participant to enjoy the activities and exercises.

Segment 1

This–Now

- Sit comfortably with your back straight and your feet pointing straight ahead.
- Close your eyes.
- Breathe normally, paying attention to each inhalation and exhalation.
- Repeat five times.
- Begin with an inhale, saying "this" to yourself.
- Exhale, saying "now" to yourself.
- Repeat 10 times, slowly.

It may be helpful to softly say, "inhale," "exhale," "this," and "now" until each participant feels comfortable with the technique.

Segment 2

Song: "Simple Gifts"

> "'Tis a gift to be simple, 'tis a gift to be free,
> 'Tis a gift to come down where we ought to be,
> And when we find ourselves in the place just right,
> 'Twill be in the valley of love and delight." (Fox, 1987)

Sing the song in its entirety before asking the participants to repeat the song line by line. When the song is completely memorized, sing it together a few more times.

Ask the participants to close their eyes while you slowly sing the song. Ask them to pay attention to the last line, "'Twill be in the valley of love and delight." What images can they visualize? Sing the song once more, and ask the participants to recapture any images the song evokes for them (e.g., a warm, sunny day; grassy fields; birds flying). How does the song make them feel? Have them describe in a few words any memories this song may evoke.

Segment 3

Bilateral Integration Exercises

Introduce the bilateral exercises by discussing the benefits of crossing the midline. Demonstrate what this means. Balance and coordination are necessary to prevent falls, and they assist us with relieving anxiety and confusion. As in the yoga postures, demonstrate how you are like a mirror image of what the participants are doing with their arms or legs in each exercise.

Bilateral Exercises 1a: Seated

Shoulder Shrugs

- Sit with your back straight and arms at your sides.

- Breathe normally.

- Lift your shoulders up toward your ears.

- Lower your shoulders, relaxing your neck.

- Repeat five times.

Large Arm Circles

- Sit with your back straight, feet pointed straight ahead.

- Breathe normally.

- Keep your right arm straight as you circle your arm clockwise in front of your body.

- Repeat three times.

- Circle your right arm counterclockwise.

- Repeat three times.

- Keep your left arm straight as you circle your arm clockwise in front of your body.

- Repeat three times.
- Circle your left arm counterclockwise.
- Repeat three times.

Elbow Stretch and Cross

- Sit with your back straight, arms at your sides.
- Clasp your hands behind your neck with your elbows out to the side.
- Exhale and bring your right elbow toward your left knee.
- Keep your head straight while gazing at your left elbow.
- Inhale and straighten your torso.
- Exhale and bring your left elbow toward your right knee.
- Keep your head straight while gazing at your right elbow.
- Inhale and straighten your torso.
- Repeat five times.

Bilateral Exercise 1b: Standing

Toe, Leg, and Arm Cross

- Standing behind your chair, use your right hand to hold on to the top of your chair.
- Stand straight with your feet together.
- Breathe normally.
- Lift your left arm straight up at your left side, shoulder level.
- Place your left foot out, shoulder width.
- Swing your left arm to the right, past your torso.
- Repeat three times.
- Swing your left foot past your right leg, toes touching the floor.

- Repeat three times.
- Swing both your left arm and left foot together.
- Repeat three times.
- Turn and face the opposite direction.
- Standing behind your chair, use your left hand to hold on to the top of your chair.
- Stand straight with your feet together.
- Breathe normally.
- Lift your right arm straight up at your right side, shoulder level.
- Place your right foot out, shoulder width.
- Swing your right arm to the left, past your torso.
- Repeat three times.
- Swing your right foot past your left leg, toes touching the floor.
- Repeat three times.
- Swing both your right arm and right foot together.
- Repeat three times.
- Incorporate the song "Simple Gifts" (Fox, 1987).
- While swinging your left arm and foot, sing in a medium tempo:

    "'Tis a gift to be simple, 'tis a gift to be free,
    'Tis a gift to come down where we ought to be."

- Turn and change directions.
- While swinging your right arm and foot, continue singing the song

    "And when we find ourselves in the place just right,
    'Twill be in the valley of love and delight."

- Repeat the movements with the song three times.

Segment 4

Simple Song, Simple Dance

Play a soft rendition of "Simple Gifts" in the background, either on audiotape or CD. The dance step is an easy two-step.

- Begin by revisiting the song "Simple Gifts" (Fox, 1987):

  "'Tis a gift to be simple, 'tis a gift to be free,
  'Tis a gift to come down where we ought to be,
  And when we find ourselves in the place just right,
  'Twill be in the valley of love and delight."

- Sing the song together a couple of times.

- Ask the participants to sing the song while you demonstrate the dance steps.

- Bring your right foot forward.

- Bring your left foot forward, next to your right foot.

- With feet together, bring your right foot back.

- Bring your left foot back, next to your right foot.

- Repeat several times, beginning with your right foot.

- Swing both arms forward and up over your head while stepping forward.

- Swing both arms down next to your body while stepping back.

- Ask participants to join you by forming a circle.

- Join hands.

- Review the dance steps without the song.

- Begin to incorporate the song with the dance steps.

Segment 5

A Simple Tea Party

The theme of this class is reinforced by arousing the senses of taste and smell. This is a time when childhood and early adult memories can be recounted. Our personal histories live inside us because we carry the blood and bones of our ancestors. They are just as much a part of us as our heartbeat and breath.

- Revisit the song "Simple Gifts" (Fox, 1987):

    "'Tis a gift to be simple, 'tis a gift to be free,
    'Tis a gift to come down where we ought to be,
    And when we find ourselves in the place just right,
    'Twill be in the valley of love and delight."

- Ask one of the participants to turn on the electric teapot.

- Pass around the basket of herbal teas.

- While the water is warming, ask each participant which tea he or she has chosen.

- Inquire if any of the participants have memories of tea parties from their youth.

- Pour the water in each cup with an herbal tea bag inside the cup.

- After the tea is ready to drink, pass around the milk, sugar, and honey.

- Invite the participants to close their eyes while they smell the aroma of the tea.

- Ask the participants if any simple delights are recalled by the smell and taste of the tea.

CLASS 3

A GRAIN OF
SAND AND A WILD FLOWER

As you did with Class 1, stay with Class 2 until the participants demonstrate a sense of completion. Over time, the
participants will become more at ease with you and the
program and will feel free to express their preferences
and opinions.

Introduce the theme of Class 3 at the end of your final
Class 2. Discuss the title of Class 3: "A Grain of Sand and
a Wild Flower." For many participants, their childhood and
a early adult years were connected to the natural world.
Without television, answering machines, and the Internet,
life brought them face to face with their earthly landscapes
and environments. As one participant stated, "In my neigh-
borhood, all of the children played outside. We would make
up our own games and build our own toys."

Segment 1

Conscious Breathing Exercise

"Breathing in, I know I am
breathing in.
"Breathing out, I know I am
breathing out."
—Thich Nhat Hanh (1991)

- Sit comfortably with your back straight and your feet pointing straight ahead.

- Close your eyes.

- Breathe normally, paying attention to each inhalation and exhalation.

- Repeat five times.

- Breathe in and say to yourself, "Breathing in, I know I am breathing in."

- Breathe out and say to yourself, "Breathing out, I know I am breathing out."

- Repeat 10 times.

Recite the exercise once before rehearsing it with the participants. Ask them to join you in reciting the words. You may want to softly say the words, "Breathing in, I know I am breathing in" as you inhale together, and say, "Breathing out, I know I am breathing out" as you exhale together for three to five repetitions.

Segment 2

Poem: "A Grain of Sand and a Wild Flower"

"To see a World in a Grain of Sand
And a Heaven in a Wild Flower,
Hold Infinity in the palm of your hand
And Eternity in an hour."
—William Blake (Kazin, 1968)

The powerful images in this poem captivate the mind and at the same time linger in a timeless realm.

With the participants' eyes closed, recite the poem, emphasizing key words and phrases from the poem: "grain of sand," "wild flower," "palm of your hand," and "eternity in an hour." After the participants have opened their eyes, ask what colors, textures, feelings, and memories came to mind.

Segment 3

Yoga Postures

Warm-Ups 2 (Seated Postures)

Head Rolls

- Place your hands in your lap.

- Relax your shoulders.

- Breathe naturally.

- Relax your head, looking straight ahead.

- Gently bend your head forward.

- Bring your head back, looking straight ahead.

- Slowly rotate your head to the left side so your ear is over your shoulder.

- Bring your head back to center.

- Slowly rotate your head to the right side so your ear is over your shoulder.

- Bring your head back to center.

- Repeat five times.

Stretch with Tie

- Hold a tie pulled tight at each end.

- Straighten your arms and place the tie on your lap.

- Maintain tension between your hands.

- Begin by raising your arms slowly, inhaling, until your arms are overhead.

- Exhale and bring your arms slowly down to your lap.

- Repeat five times.

- Incorporate the following poem:

> "To see a World in a Grain of Sand
> And a Heaven in a Wild Flower,
> Hold Infinity in the palm of your hand
> And Eternity in an hour."
> —William Blake (Kazin, 1968)

- Repeat the poem two times.

Seated Leg and Arm Postures 2

Side Stretch

- Sit with your feet slightly apart.
- Inhale and raise your arms out to your sides, shoulder height.
- Exhale and bend toward the left, keeping your arms and back straight.
- Inhale and return to center.
- Exhale and bend toward the right, keeping your arms and back straight.
- Inhale and return to center.
- Repeat three times.

Knee Squeeze

- Sit with your feet slightly apart.
- Exhale completely.
- Inhale and lift your right leg with both hands under your knee.
- Gently pull your knee toward your chest, tucking your head in.
- Exhale and release.
- Inhale and lift your left leg with both hands under your knee.

- Gently pull your knee toward your chest, tucking your head in.
- Exhale and release.
- Repeat three times.

Standing Chair Postures 2

Side Leg Lifts

- With your right hand, hold on to the top of your chair.
- Stand straight with your feet together.
- Place your left hand on your hip.
- Exhale completely.
- Inhale and lift your left leg up to the side.
- Exhale and lower your leg.
- Repeat three times.
- Turn and face the opposite direction.
- With your left hand, hold on to the top of your chair.
- Place your right hand on your hip.
- Exhale completely.
- Inhale and lift your right leg up to the side.
- Exhale and lower your leg.
- Repeat three times.

Chair Twist

- With your right hand, hold on to the top of your chair.
- Stand straight with your feet together.
- Exhale completely.
- Inhale and lift your left arm over your head.
- Exhale and slowly twist your torso to the right.

- Inhale and twist your torso back to center.
- Lower your left arm.
- Repeat three times.
- Turn and face the opposite direction.
- With your left hand, hold on to the top of your chair.
- Stand straight with your feet together.
- Exhale completely.
- Inhale and lift your right arm over your head.
- Exhale and slowly twist your torso to the left.
- Inhale and twist your torso back to center.
- Lower your right arm.
- Repeat three times.

Segment 4

Poetry and Music

Begin this segment by demonstrating how each rhythm instrument is played. Ask the participants to pick an instrument.

- Allow each participant to become acquainted with the instrument he or she chooses.

- When the participants feel comfortable with the instruments they have selected, lay them aside.

- Recite the following poem together:

> "To see a World in a Grain of Sand
> And a Heaven in a Wild Flower,
> Hold Infinity in the palm of your hand
> And Eternity in an hour."
> —William Blake (Kazin, 1968)

- Ask the participants to listen while you recite the poem with a distinct cadence, emphasizing the words *see, world, grain, sand, heaven, flower, infinity, palm, hand, eternity,* and *hour.*

- Together, recite the poem slowly with an accent on the emphasized words.

- Demonstrate how each instrument is played when the accented words are said.

- Recite the poem and play the instruments together.

- When the poem and rhythm are synchronized, play three more rounds.

Segment 5

A Grain of Sand and a Wild Flower

The poet e.e. cummings wrote as the first line of a poem, "Since feeling is first" (Firmage, 1985), referring to how we perceive the world through our senses before our minds begin to process information. In this activity, the senses of touch and smell awaken each participant's ability to concentrate and retrieve memories from the past.

- Recite the following poem together:

> "To see a World in a Grain of Sand
> And a Heaven in a Wild Flower,
> Hold Infinity in the palm of your hand
> And Eternity in an hour."
> —William Blake (Kazin, 1968)

- Invite the participants to feel the sand with their fingers.

- Ask each participant to notice the texture of the sand.

- Let each participant pick a flower from the vase.

- Ask the participants to pay attention to the scent of their flowers.

- Ask the participants to identify the colors and textures associated with their flowers.

- Recite the Blake poem together.

- Have the participants close their eyes and think of the sand and their flowers.

- Ask each participant what stands out in his or her mind (e.g., color, scent, texture).

- Ask the participants to recall any memories that arise from this experience.

SWEET BETSY'S ANIMAL FAIR

The last example for a Movement with Meaning class draws from our collective American folklore. It has been my experience that songs such as "Sweet Betsy from Pike" conjure up many childhood memories. One participant brought an early 1920s volume of favorite American folk songs to a Movement with Meaning class. Each participant picked a song, and for one entire class we sang the songs from the book. At the end of the class, I asked the participants if they would like to agree to use one of the songs for a future class. The participants chose "My Bonnie Lies Over the Ocean." I had my homework to do. I wove the theme of crossing the ocean through each segment of the class. The participants brought seashells, artifacts from Hawaii, poems, and photographs depicting seaside vacations from their childhood and early adult years.

Segment 1

Soft Breathing

- Sit comfortably with your back straight and your feet pointing straight ahead.
- Close your eyes.
- Breathe normally, paying attention to each inhalation and exhalation.
- Repeat five times.
- Take a deep breath and repeat to yourself, "soft belly."
- Exhale and relax.
- Repeat 10 times.
- Breathe normally again.

For the first three or four breaths, you may want to softly say "soft belly" with each inhalation to help the participants concentrate on their stomach muscles.

Song: "Sweet Betsy from Pike"

"Oh, don't your remember Sweet Betsy from Pike?
Who crossed the big mountains with her lover Ike.
With two yoke of oxen, a big yaller dog,
A tall Shanghai rooster, and one spotted hog."

—"Sweet Betsy from Pike" (Fox, 1987)

Most of the participants are familiar with this folk song, so it is likely that you will need to sing it only once in its entirety. Sing the song together until a natural harmony and cadence is established.

Ask the participants to close their eyes while you slowly sing the song, requesting that they pay attention to the images. Have them focus on the colors, season, and images that Betsy, Ike, and their animal friends bring forth as the participants visualize this fun-spirited folk song.

Segment 3

Bilateral Integration Exercises

Take your time, demonstrating each bilateral exercise slowly. Pay attention to the natural rhythm each exercise evokes. Emphasize the importance of maintaining balance and coordination to prevent falls and relieve anxiety and confusion.

Bilateral Exercises 2a: Seated

Body Stretch

- Sit straight, with your back slightly away from your chair.

- Place both feet apart, a little wider than the width of your hips.

- Interlace your fingers.

- Inhale as you straighten your arms and raise them over your head.

- Exhale and lower your arms to shoulder height with your fingers interlaced.

- Inhale and move your arms to the right with your fingers interlaced.

- Exhale and come back to center.

- Inhale and move your arms to the left with your fingers interlaced.

- Exhale and come back to center.

- Interlace your fingers, inhale, and straighten your arms and raise them over your head.

- Exhale, lowering your head, torso, and arms to the floor.

- Inhale and slowly raise your head, torso, and arms.
- Release your fingers, and place your hands on your knees.
- Repeat three times.

Ankle–Knee Slaps

- Sit straight, with your feet slightly apart.
- Cross your right ankle over your left knee.
- With your left hand, slap your ankle, then your knee.
- Repeat three times.
- Cross your left ankle over your right knee.
- With your right hand, slap your ankle, then your knee.
- Repeat three times.
- Incorporate the song "Sweet Betsy from Pike" (Fox, 1987).
- Cross your right ankle over your left knee, and slap your ankle and knee in tempo with the first two lines:

  "Oh, don't you remember Sweet Betsy from Pike?
  Who crossed the big mountains with her lover Ike."

- Cross your left ankle over your right knee, and slap your ankle and knee in tempo with the last two lines:

  "With two yoke of oxen, a big yaller dog,
  A tall Shanghai rooster, and one spotted hog."

- Repeat three times.

Bilateral Exercises 2b: Standing

Cross-Over

- Stand facing the back of your chair.
- Hold on to the top of the chair with your right hand in front of your left leg.

- Straighten your right arm.
- Breathe normally.
- Lift your left arm in a circular motion, passing it over your head.
- Place your left hand on the top of the chair in front of your right leg.
- Straighten your left arm.
- Lift your right arm in a circular motion, passing it over your head.
- Place your right hand on the top of the chair in front of your left leg.
- Repeat the sequence five times.

Scissor Leg Lifts

- With your right hand, hold on to the top of the chair.
- Stand straight with your feet together.
- Place your left hand on your hip.
- Inhale and lift your left leg to the side.
- Exhale and lower your left leg.
- Cross your left leg over your right leg, toes touching the floor.
- Inhale and lift your left leg to the side.
- Exhale and lower your left leg.
- Cross your left leg behind your right leg, toes touching the floor.
- Repeat three times.
- Turn and face the opposite direction.
- With your left hand, hold on to the top of the chair.
- Stand straight with your feet together.

- Place your right hand on your hip.

- Inhale and lift your right leg to the side.

- Exhale and lower your right leg.

- Cross your right leg over your left leg, toes touching the floor.

- Inhale and lift your right leg to the side.

- Exhale and lower your right leg.

- Cross your right leg behind your left leg, toes touching the floor.

- Repeat three times.

Segment 4

Circle Dance with Betsy

This dance can be accompanied with recorded music or simply with an *a capella* song. The tempo is a steady four- or eight-count beat, depending on the group's level of motor development.

- Begin by revisiting "Sweet Betsy from Pike" (Fox, 1987):

  "Oh, don't you remember Sweet Betsy from Pike?
  Who crossed the big mountains with her lover Ike.
  With two yoke of oxen, a big yaller dog,
  A tall Shanghai rooster, and one spotted hog."

- Sing the song together a couple of times.

- Ask the participants to sing the song while you demonstrate the circle dance.

- Step in to a count of four, lifting your arms.

- Step out to a count of four, lowering your arms.

- Circle to the right to a count of four.

- Circle to the left to a count of four.

- Ask the participants to join you in forming a circle.

- Join hands.

- Review the steps without the song.

- Begin to incorporate the song with the circle dance.

Segment 5

Sweet Betsy's Animal Fair

At the end of Class 4, write a note asking each participant to bring in a photograph of a beloved pet, either from childhood or from any time in his or her adult life. Bring a variety of stuffed but realistic-looking animals or laminated animal pictures to class. Include a dog, pig, and rooster to reinforce the animals in the song.

- Begin this segment by singing "Sweet Betsy from Pike" (Fox, 1987):

  "Oh don't you remember Sweet Betsy from Pike?
  Who crossed the big mountains with her lover Ike.
      With two yoke of oxen, a big yaller dog,
      A tall Shanghai rooster, and one spotted hog."

- Ask the participants to pick a stuffed animal or laminated animal picture.

- Invite the participants to share any adventures they had with a childhood pet or farm animal.

- Introduce a photograph of a special animal in your life.

- Ask the participants if they would like to share a photograph of a favorite pet.

- Give each participant the opportunity to reminisce about their beloved pet with a short story, with a particular characteristic they treasure, or just by passing around a photograph.

EPILOGUE

The individuals with whom I have worked have exhibited extraordinary resilience when given the opportunity to thrive in the present, connected to the essential core of their being. Time and time again, I have witnessed triumph amidst tragedy.

Individuals with Alzheimer's disease have taught me that nothing is what it appears to be on the surface. This world is filled with mystery and hidden treasures. I was pleasantly forced to become a detective, investigating the corridors of the Alzheimer's mind. The multisensory activities acted as searchlights as I ventured through the cool mist, providing me with a deeper insight into the profound experiences of the person with Alzheimer's disease. The activities also offered me a vital opportunity to look behind the mask of Alzheimer's disease and stop my inner chatter—to wait and listen. I had to give up any dogmatic certainty and direct my attention to the more subtle forms of metaphorical and symbolic language.

My intuitive nature evolved through this process, and I was able to abandon the notion of time as simply a linear phenomenon. I journeyed into the realm of "between" worlds with these remarkable individuals. I had to tune in and make my body a good receptor. As my senses awoke, I began to venture not only on an educational journey but on a spiritual sojourn as well. The participants asked me to be *present*, and thereby, to see the sacred in the ordinary.

For those of us who are fortunate enough to work in the field of dementia care, I can think of no better way to express our gratitude than with these words from the Sufi poet, Rumi (Ryan, 1994):

"Let the beauty we love be what we do.
There are a hundred ways to kneel and kiss the ground."

Appendix A

Suggested Readings

Bayley, J. (1999). *Elegy for Iris.* New York: Picador USA.

Bell, V., & Troxel, D. (1997). *The best friends approach to Alzheimer's care.* Baltimore: Health Professions Press.

Brackey, J. (2000). *Creating moments of joy for the person with Alzheimer's or dementia.* West Lafayette, IN: Purdue University Press.

Christensen, A. (1995). *20-minute yoga workouts.* New York: Random House.

Clair, A.A. (1996). *Therapeutic uses of music with older adults.* Baltimore: Health Professions Press.

Cordrey, C. (1994). *Hidden treasures: Music and memory activities for people with Alzheimer's.* Mt. Airy, MD: Elder-Song Publications.

Farhi, D. (1996). *The breathing book.* New York: Henry Holt & Company.

Higbee, K. (1996). *Your memory: How it works and how to improve it.* New York: Marlowe.

Khalsa, D.S., & Stauth, C. (1997). *Brain longevity: The breakthrough medical program that improves your mind and memory.* New York: Warner Books.

Kirkland, K., & McIlveen, H. (1999). *Full circle: Spiritual therapy for the elderly.* Binghamton, NY: Haworth Press.

Kuhn, D. (1999). *Alzheimer's early stages: First steps in caring and treatment.* Alameda, CA: Hunter House.

Lustbader, W. (1991). *Counting on kindness: The dilemmas of dependency.* New York: Free Press.

Marcels, N. (2001). *Home sanctuary: Practical ways to create a spiritually fulfilling environment.* Chicago: Contemporary Press.

Nissenboim, S., & Vroman, C. (1997). *The positive interactions program of activities for people with Alzheimer's disease.* Baltimore: Health Professions Press.

Roberts, E., & Amidon, E. (Eds.). (1991). *Earth prayers from around the world: 365 prayers, poems, and invocations for honoring the earth.* New York: HarperCollins.

Rybarczyk, B., & Bellg, A. (1997). *Listening to life stories: A new approach to stress intervention in health care.* New York: Springer.

Sacks, O. (1985). *The man who mistook his wife for a hat and other clinical tales.* New York: Simon & Schuster.

Shankle, W.R., & Amen, D.G. (2004). *Preventing Alzheimer's: Prevent, detect, diagnose, treat, and even halt Alzheimer's disease and other causes of memory loss.* New York: G.P. Putnam's Sons.

Small, G. (2002). *The memory bible.* New York: Hyperion.

Snyder, L. (1999). *Speaking our minds: Personal reflections from individuals with Alzheimer's disease.* New York: W.H. Freeman.

Watson, B. (1996). *Music, movement, mind, and body: Exercises for people suffering from Alzheimer's disease and related disorders.* Forest Knolls, CA: Elder Books.

Appendix B

Resource Catalogs

Alzheimer's Sensory Stimulation Resources

Geriatric Resources
Telephone: 800-359-0390
Website: http://www.geriatric-resources.com

Attainment Company
Telephone: 800-327-4269
Website: http://www.AttainmentCompany.com

Creative Arts Therapy Resources

MMB Music
Telephone: 800-543-3771
Website: http://www.mmbmusic.com

ElderSong Publications
Telephone: 800-397-0533
Website: http://www.eldersong.com

West Music
Telephone: 800-397-9378
Website: http://www.westmusic.com

Older Adult Mental Health and Wellness Resources

Wellness Reproductions & Publishing
Telephone: 800-669-9208
Website: http://www.wellness-resources.com

Reminiscence Resources

BiFolkal Production
Telephone: 800-568-5357
Website: http://www.bifolkal.org

Elder Books
The Alzheimer's Bookshelf
Telephone: 800-909-2673
Website: http://www.elderbooks.com

The Alzheimer's Store
Telephone: 800-752-3238
Website: http://www.alzstore.com

References

Albrecht, S. (2003, Spring). Activity design for individuals with mild to moderate Alzheimer's dementia. *Activities Directors' Quarterly for Alzheimer's & Other Dementia Patients, 4*(2), 1–7.

Aldridge, D. (1994). Alzheimer's disease: Rhythm, timing and music as therapy. *Biomedicine and Pharamacotherapy, 48*(7), 275–281.

Alzheimer's Association. (1992). *Environment.* Chicago: Author.

Arst, C. (1997, October 6). Songs that lead down memory lane. *Business Week,* 75.

Bakker, R. (2003, Spring). Sensory loss, dementia, and environments. *Generations, 27*(1), 46–51.

Bayley, J. (1999). *Elegy for Iris.* New York: Picador USA.

Bell, V., & Troxel, D. (1997). *The best friends approach to Alzheimer's care.* Baltimore: Health Professions Press.

Berg, K.D., & Kairy, D. (2003, Winter). Falls and fall-related injuries: Balance interventions to prevent falls. *Generations, 26*(4), 75–78.

Berry, W. (1992). *Fidelity: Five stories.* New York: Pantheon.

Brackey, J. (2000). *Creating moments of joy for the person with Alzheimer's or dementia.* West Lafayette, IN: Purdue University Press.

Brawley, E. (1997). *Designing for Alzheimer's disease: Strategies for creating better care environments.* New York: John Wiley & Sons.

Burns, A., Byrne, J., & Ballard, C. (2002). Sensory stimulation in dementia: An effective option for managing behavioural problems. *British Medical Journal, 325,* 1312–1313.

Burns, T., McCarten, J., Adler, G., Bauer, M., & Kuskowski, M.A. (2004, January/February). Effects of repetitive work on maintaining function in Alzheimer's disease patients. *American Journal of Alzheimer's Disease & Other Dementia, 19*(1), 39–44.

Campbell, J. (with Moyers, B.). (1988). *The power of myth.* New York: Doubleday.

Chaucer, G. (1894). *Chaucer's Canterbury tales.* New York: Macmillan and Co.

Coste, J. (2003). *Learning to speak Alzheimer's: A groundbreaking approach for everyone dealing with the disease.* New York: Houghton Mifflin.

Coulter, H.D. (2001). *Anatomy of hatha yoga: A manual for student, teachers, and practitioners.* Honesdale, PA: Body and Breath.

Dennison, P., & Dennison, G. (1994). *Brain gym.* Ventura, CA: The Education Kinesiology Foundation.

Drabben-Thiemann, G., et al. (2002). The effect of brain gym on cognitive performance of Alzheimer's patients. *Brain Gym Journal.* Retrieved January 29, 2004, from http://www.braingym.org/alzheimer's.html

Erickson, L.M., & Leide, K. (1992). Touch, taste and smell the memories. *Activities, Adaptation, and Aging, 16*(3), 25–39.

Farhi, D. (1996). *The breathing book.* New York: Henry Holt & Company.

Fazio, S., Seman, D., & Stansell, J. (1999). *Rethinking Alzheimer's care.* Baltimore: Health Professions Press.

Feil, N. (2002). *The validation breakthrough: Simple techniques for communicating with people with Alzheimer's-type dementia* (2nd ed.). Baltimore: Health Professions Press.

Firmage, G. (Ed.). (1985). Complete Poems: 1904–1962 by e.e. cummings. New York: Liveright Publishing Corporation.

Folstein, M.F. (2001). *Mini-mental state examination (MMSE): Clinical guide.* Lutz, FL: Psychological Assessment Resources.

Fox, D. (Ed.). (1987). *Go in and out the window: An illustrated songbook for young children.* New York: The Metropolitan Museum of Art & Henry Holt and Company.

Gardner, H. (Ed.). (1973). *The new Oxford book of English verse.* New York: Oxford University Press.

Graham, M. (1991). *Blood memory.* New York: Doubleday.

Gross, T. (2002, January 29). Interview with Rudolf Tanzi. *Fresh Air* (National Public Radio). Philadelphia: WHYY.

Higbee, K. (1996). *Your memory: How it works and how to improve it.* New York: Marlowe.

Hill, H. (1999, May). Dance therapy and communication in dementia. *Signpost to Older People and Mental Health Matters, 4*(1). Retrieved January 29, 2004, from http://www.phewartscompany.co.uk/dementia.html

Karp, A., Paillard-Borg, S., Wang, H.X., Silverstein, M., Winblad, B., & Fratiglioni, L. (2004, July). Mental, physical and social components in common leisure activities in old age in relation to dementia. *Neurobiology of Aging, 25*(S2), 313.

Kazin, A. (1968). *The portable Blake.* New York: Viking Press.

Khalsa, D.S., & Stauth, C. (1997). *Brain longevity: The breakthrough medical program that improves your mind and memory.* New York: Warner Books.

Kingsolver, B. (1989). *Homeland and other stories.* New York: HarperPerennial.

Kirkland, K., & McIlveen, H. (1999). *Full circle: Spiritual therapy for the elderly.* Binghamton, NY: Haworth Press.

Kotre, J. (1999–2000, Winter). Reasons to grow old: Meaning in later life. Generativity and the gift of meaning. *Generations, 23*(4), 65–70.

Kuhn, D. (1999). *Alzheimer's early stages: First steps in caring and treatment.* Alameda, CA: Hunter House.

Mathews, R., Clair, A., & Kosloski, K. (2001, November/December). Keeping the beat: Use of rhythmic music during exercise activities for the elderly with dementia. *American Journal of Alzheimer's Disease and Other Dementia,* 377–380.

Mayes, F. (1996). *Under the Tuscan sun.* New York: Broadway Books.

Mehta, S., Mehta, M., & Mehta, S. (1990). *Yoga: The Iyengar way.* New York: Alfred A. Knopf.

Muir, J. (1979). *My first summer in the Sierra.* New York: Houghton Mifflin.

Paige, H.W. (1999). Echoes of a lost Sunday. *Early Alzheimer's: An international newsletter on dementia, 2*(1), 1, 10.

Pettersson, A.F., Engardt, M., & Wahlund, L.O. (2002). Activity level and balance in subjects with mild Alzheimer's disease. *Dementia Geriatric Cognitive Disorders, 13*(4), 213–216.

Rodgers, A.B. (2004, October). *2003 progress report on Alzheimer's disease.* Bethesda, MD: U.S. National Institutes of Health, National Institute on Aging.

Ryan, M. (Ed.). (1994). *A grateful heart: Daily blessings for the evening meal from Buddha to the Beatles.* Emeryville, CA: Conari Press.

Sacks, O. (1985). *The man who mistook his wife for a hat and other clinical tales.* New York: Simon & Schuster.

Schmall, V., Cleland, M., & Sturdevant, M. (2000). *The caregiver helpbook.* Portland, OR: Legacy Health System.

Shankle, W.R., & Amen, D.G. (2004). *Preventing Alzheimer's: Prevent, detect, diagnose, treat, and even halt Alzheimer's disease and other causes of memory loss.* New York: G.P. Putnam's Sons.

Small, G. (2002). *The memory bible.* New York: Hyperion.

Suhr, J., Anderson, S., & Tranel, D. (1999). Progressive muscle relaxation in the management of behavioral disturbance in Alzheimer' disease. *Neuropsychological Rehabilitation, 9,* B1–44.

Tappen, R.M. (1997). *Interventions for Alzheimer's disease: A caregiver's complete reference.* Baltimore: Health Professions Press.

Thich Nhat Hanh. (1992). *Peace is every step.* New York: Bantam.

Todd, M.L., & Higginson, T.W. (Eds.). (1982). *Complete poems of Emily Dickinson.* New York: Crown.

Walter, J. (Ed.). (1885). *George Eliot's life as related in her letters and journals.* New York: Harper & Brothers.

Whitman, W. (1855). *Leaves of grass.* New York: Doubleday, Page & Company.

Williams, T. (1972). *Memoirs.* New York: Doubleday & Company.

Woods, B. (1999, Fall). State of the art for practice in dementia: The person in dementia care. *Generations, 23*(3), 35–39.

Yale, R. (1995). *Developing support groups for individuals with early-stage Alzheimer's disease: Planning, implementation, and evaluation.* Baltimore: Health Professions Press.

Credits

Date Due

DEC 15 2010		
JUN 01 2012		
JAN 31 2012		